Psoriasis - Recent Advances in Diagnosis and Treatment

Edited by Pierre Vereecken

Published in London, United Kingdom

Psoriasis - Recent Advances in Diagnosis and Treatment
http://dx.doi.org/10.5772/intechopen.1000431
Edited by Pierre Vereecken

Contributors
Aleena Boby, Amanda Krenitsky, Angeliki-Victoria Roussaki-Schulze, Anthony P. Gulotta, Ariel T. Kidron, Celenkosini Thembelenkosini Nxumalo, Efterpi Zafiriou, Emmanouil Karampinis, Km. Reena, Lalit Singh, Michael F. Land, Mokgadi Makgobole, Nicole Natarelli, Nomakhosi Mpofana, Pavitra Pillay, Pierre Vereecken, Ritesh Kumar Tiwari, Shaliz Aflatooni

First published in London, United Kingdom, 2024 by IntechOpen
IntechOpen is the global imprint of INTECHOPEN LIMITED, registered in England and Wales, registration number: 11086078, 167-169 Great Portland Street, London, W1W 5PF, United Kingdom

British Library Cataloguing-in-Publication Data
A catalogue record for this book is available from the British Library

Additional hard and PDF copies can be obtained from orders@intechopen.com

Psoriasis - Recent Advances in Diagnosis and Treatment
Edited by Pierre Vereecken
p. cm.
Print ISBN 978-1-83769-380-1
Online ISBN 978-1-83769-379-5
eBook (PDF) ISBN 978-1-83769-381-8

For EU product safety concerns:
IN TECH d.o.o., Prolaz Marije Krucifikse Kozulić 3, 51000 Rijeka, Croatia,
info@intechopen.com or visit our website at intechopen.com.

Meet the editor

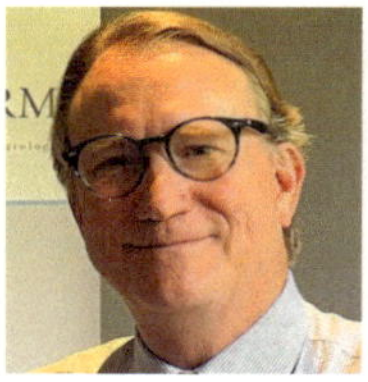

Dr. Pierre Vereecken, MD, Ph.D., is qualified in dermatology (general, aesthetic, and corrective) as well as in cutaneous oncology. He studied medicine at the Université libre de Bruxelles, Belgium (1991, ULB). After working for the Belgian Army and the United Nations Protection Force, he obtained a Ph.D. with a thesis on the biology and progression of cutaneous malignant melanoma in 2008. From 2007 to 2011, he was the head of the Department of Dermatology, University Hospital, Brussels. In 2011, Dr. Vereecken created Cliderm (Clinics in Dermatology), an international network of dermatologists, as well as the European Institute for Dermatology Practice and Research, a multifaceted structure that aims to promote clinical dermatology and dermatology research within the European Union.

Contents

Preface **IX**

Section 1
Treating the Psoriasis Patients with a New Paradigm **1**

Chapter 1 **3**
Introductory Chapter: New Challenges for Practionners, New Roads for Patients
by Pierre Vereecken

Section 2
Clues to Better Recognize the Psoriasis Patients and Understand Their Life Stories **7**

Chapter 2 **9**
Psoriasis: Clinical Features and Its Impact on Quality of Life
by Nomakhosi Mpofana, Mokgadi Makgobole, Celenkosini Thembelenkosini Nxumalo and Pavitra Pillay

Chapter 3 **35**
Psoriasis and Exposome: Unveiling the Inner and the External Contributors of Psoriasis Disease
by Efterpi Zafiriou, Emmanouil Karampinis and Angeliki-Victoria Roussaki-Schulze

Chapter 4 **55**
Psychosocial Burden and Psychological Interventions for Patients with Psoriasis
by Nicole Natarelli, Aleena Boby, Shaliz Aflatooni and Amanda Krenitsky

Section 3
Daring New Roads **69**

Chapter 5 **71**
Biologics: Beyond the Basics
by Ariel T. Kidron, Anthony P. Gulotta and Michael F. Land

Chapter 6 85
Perspective Chapter: Role of Curcumin in the Management of Rheumatoid Arthritis and Psoriatic Arthritis
by Km. Reena, Lalit Singh and Ritesh Kumar Tiwari

Preface

Psoriasis is a remarkably common condition, yet many patients receive inadequate care.

Many psoriasis patients are not given the opportunity to fully express their situation or describe how their condition profoundly impacts their quality of life. It is disheartening to witness so many patients going without thorough examinations, despite evidence indicating that psoriasis extends beyond mere skin affliction. Indeed, there is a litany of associated conditions, such as depression, psoriatic arthritis, obesity, hypertension, metabolic syndrome, diabetes, and more.

As such, there is undoubtedly a need to confirm that psoriasis is underdiagnosed, neglected, and inadequately treated. It is therefore imperative for practitioners to embrace multidisciplinary care to better identify and manage patients. We must strive to improve patient knowledge of the condition and empower patients to mitigate the impact of psoriasis on their health and overall well-being, a concept now termed patient empowerment.

This book provides new insights into the identification and management of psoriasis and encourages a holistic approach to patient care.

Pierre Vereecken
Cliderm Medical Office,
Brussels, Belgium

Section 1

Treating the Psoriasis Patients with a New Paradigm

Chapter 1

Introductory Chapter: New Challenges for Practionners, New Roads for Patients

Pierre Vereecken

1. Psoriasis: A common multifaceted disease

Psoriasis is an autoinflammatory skin disease that can be defined by an accelerated rate of epidermal turnover including hyperproliferation and defective maturation of epidermal keratinocytes [1]. It is a chronic disease that first occurs more frequently in the second and third decades of life but can be observed at any age. Its prevalence reaches 2% in northern countries, North America, and Europe, probably less in southern countries. It seems important to review what the practitioners can find in psoriatic patients, from the classical chronic plaque psoriasis, with well-demarcated thickened and scaly plaques, often symmetrically distributed, to the other presentations namely guttate psoriasis, flexural or inverse psoriasis, palms and soles hyperkeratosis, nails distorted by thimble pits, nail plate thickening, and detachment. Recognizing all these signs allows rapid relief for the patient and surely the best support. Too many patients will still come lately after years of suffering.

2. Behind the skin lesions

In up to 30% of patients with psoriasis, arthritis can be associated, a seronegative for rheumatoid factor. The prevalence of arthritis among psoriatic patients emphasizes the need for a multidisciplinary approach with assessment of both skin and joints by general practitioners, dermatologists, and rheumatologists.

Psoriasis is also associated with comorbidities such as Crohn's disease, obesity, diabetes, hypertension, and even cancer. Moreover, studies found higher degrees of depression in patients with a greater percentage of their skin affected with psoriasis. This is one more proof that multidisciplinarity is important in our daily practices. According to the WHO, the management of psoriasis does not only correspond to the treatment of skin or joint lesions but also deals with these different comorbidities [2].

3. New roads

Much is known about the epidemiology of psoriasis, but the interplay between the disease itself, the effects of the treatments, and the behavior of patients should be better investigated [3].

We have to recognize that our purpose is not only to explore all the fields of this frequent disease and to give to readers an exhaustive material but well to provide very important and practical aspects for all practitioners following psoriatic patients. This current book claims to be a practical and perspective tool.

Because most patients will not be free of disease for the rest of their lives, biological therapies are the most important information regarding a new therapeutic option [4]. These targeted and tailored therapies are able to modulate the immunity of patients and enable to define of new therapeutic aims: proportions of patients achieving clearance or near clearance are high, with excellent outcomes and patient satisfaction. Cost-effectiveness studies remain important to define the position in the therapeutic strategy. This strategy emphasizes now the concept of "hit hard and hit early" which means that every practitioner has to recognize all forms of psoriasis and to rapidly treat them with a tailored approach. Biological treatments could take a major place in the treatment of patients with psoriasis since the option could be to reduce and to space out the doses.

On the other side, there is an effort to find new treatments and other approaches than the "classical" evidence-based therapy. Many patients ask for these new and other approaches. There are more proofs of evidence that supports to explain that curcumin should help patients for instance presenting with arthritis. Curcumin is a phytopolyphenol pigment isolated from the plant *Curcuma longa* known for its anti-inflammatory properties as a result of the inhibition of cyclooxygenases (COX inhibition). It also disrupts cell signal transduction by different mechanisms including inhibition of protein kinase C. The idea is not to forget this traditional Indian spice and to remember that many therapies came directly or indirectly from perennial plants. Of course, more investigations are necessary to bring evidence-based proof and to investigate other new roads.

By the way, many studies underline the effect of the environment on patients and their diseases. This will help the patients to choose a well-balanced lifestyle, making them actors and decision-makers. This is surely the beginning of the idea of "patient empowerment" which changes the paradigm of medical approach. If the patients recognize triggering factors, the medical team will help them control their impacts on the natural history of their diseases. Studies on the impact of psoriasis have corroborated clinicians' feeling that psoriasis has a major impact on social and psychological functioning [5]. It is one more argument to regularly assess a patient's quality of life, not only by asking the patient "How are you?" but by using a multidimensional model, such as the Dermatology Life Quality Index (DLQI). No matter how much or little of the skin is involved, patients can experience deep effects from the physical, mental, or social point of view.

There is a lack of long-term studies on patients with severe chronic plaque psoriasis, despite the fact that most of the treatments show good evidence of risk of harm and side effects from most of the treatments, such as skin cancer for phototherapy, cutaneous atrophy from chronic dermocorticosteroids use, hepatic fibrosis and myelosuppression from methotrexate, renal impairment and hypertension from ciclosporin, teratogenicity from systemic retinoids, paradoxical effects or tuberculosis reactivation from biological therapies. These facts are a reminder to focus on the future of new therapies and to help the patients to control their own lives. A balance must always be found between patients' individual perceptions, constraint and side effects of the treatments.

This book will give readers, whatever the specialty of the practitioner, the opportunity to consider differently the psoriatic patient, because the patient needs more than pharmacological treatment.

Author details

Pierre Vereecken
Cliderm Medical Office, Belgium

*Address all correspondence to: dr.vereecken@dermatologist.be

References

[1] CEM G, Amstrong AW, Gudjonsson JE, JNWN B. Psoriasis. Lancet. 2021;**397**(10281):1301-1315

[2] Management of psoriasis as a systemic disease: What is the evidence. The British Journal of Dermatology. 2020;**182**(4):840-848

[3] Ujiie H, Rosmarin D, Schön MP, et al. Unmet medical needs in chronic, non-communicable inflammatory skin diseases. Frontiers in Medicine (Lausanne). 2022;**9**:875492. DOI: 10.3389/fmed.2022.875492

[4] Kim HJ, Lebwohl MG. Biologics and psoriasis: The beat goes on. Dermatologic Clinics. 2019;**37**(1):29-36

[5] Langley RG, Krueger GG, Griffiths CE. Psoriasis: Epidemiology, clinical features, and quality of life. Annals of the Rheumatic Diseases. Mar 2005;**64**(Suppl 2):ii18-23. discussion ii24-5. DOI: 10.1136/ard.2004.033217

Section 2

Clues to Better Recognize the Psoriasis Patients and Understand Their Life Stories

Chapter 2

Psoriasis: Clinical Features and Its Impact on Quality of Life

Nomakhosi Mpofana, Mokgadi Makgobole, Celenkosini Thembelenkosini Nxumalo and Pavitra Pillay

Abstract

Psoriasis is a chronic, papulo-squamous, non-infectious, immune-mediated, and inflammatory skin disorder clinically characterized by erythematous sharply demarcated papules and rounded plaques covered by silvery micaceous scales. It is associated with comorbidities such as psoriatic arthritis, depression, obesity, and cardiovascular disease. Psoriasis can also be a source of self and social rejection, thus contributing to stigmatization, alienation, and a decrease in the quality of life (QoL). Due to its complex pathogenesis, a holistic approach is necessary when treating psoriasis. In addition to treating physical symptoms, the patient's psychological and emotional health should be highly considered to help individuals cope with stigma. Likewise, an increased social awareness of psoriasis may contribute to a better understanding of the disease. Alternative stress management therapies such as spa therapies using dead sea mud and or balneotherapy, yoga, and aromatherapy may be effective in stress management to improve overall well-being and QoL.

Keywords: psoriasis, quality of life, stigmatization, therapy, treatment

1. Introduction

Psoriasis is a chronic, recurrent, autoimmune-mediated, and inflammatory skin disease characterized by distinct demarcated erythematous plaques with whitish scales [1–4]. It affects about 3% of the world's population which varies according to regions [5]. It predominantly involves the skin and joints, and it affects all genders equally [6]. Beyond the physical appearance of psoriasis, the skin disease can evoke an extensive emotional and psychological effect on patients which can result in poor self-esteem and increased stress affecting interpersonal relationships and social functioning [6].

The most prevalent form is vulgar psoriasis, which accounts for more than 80% of all psoriasis cases [7, 8]. In addition to plaque psoriasis, there are other clinical forms, such as flexural or inverse psoriasis, and these are characterized by red scales with a shiny appearance and can occasionally be mistaken for seborrheic dermatitis due to specific localization and often greasy scales [8, 9]. General psoriasis, pustular, inverse, and guttate psoriasis are less common forms of psoriasis with erythroderma, a severe condition that can develop from any type of psoriasis [9].

The pathologic process of psoriasis is multifactorial and involves dysregulated inflammation and strong genetic associations [6]. Approximately a third of patients with psoriasis have a first-degree relative with the skin condition [10]. External factors such as environmental factors, changes in season, a dry environment, sun exposure, humidity, cold, and heat can aggravate skin disease [1, 2].

When comparing psoriatic with uninvolved skin, the histological examination of chronic psoriasis plaques is distinguished by typical changes in both the dermis and epidermis [11, 12]. In the epidermis, there is hyperproliferation of keratinocytes, which leads to epidermal thickening, the elongated rete ridges that form fingerlike protrusions into the dermis. The granular layer of the epidermis becomes either reduced or missing. The epidermis becomes infiltrated by neutrophils and activated $CD8^+$ T lymphocytes.

The epidermal hyperplastic changes are associated with low expression of keratins K1 and K10, which are keratinocyte differentiation markers. There is also loss of the granular cell layer, hyperkeratosis with para-keratosis (retention of nuclei in stratum corneum cells), elongated rete ridges, the presence of micro-pustules of Kogoj and micro-abscesses of Munro as well as dilated vessels in the dermal papillae; however, the keratinocytes in the hair follicle are unaffected [2, 8, 10–12]. In the dermis, an inflammatory infiltrate composed of lymphocytes, macrophages, mast cells, and neutrophils is observed. Elongated and dilated blood vessels in the dermal papillae are caused by the increase of vascular endothelial growth factor (VEGF), as it has been shown that VEGF serum levels correlate with the clinical severity of psoriasis [8]. The presence of cytokines, dendritic cells, and T lymphocytes in psoriasis prompted the development of biological therapies [10]. Recent studies which were conducted both in mice and humans identified the IL-23/Th17 axis as a major factor in the pathogenesis of psoriasis [13, 14].

Treatment can range from topical to systemic, and the treatment choice depends on the form and severity of the disease, with biological therapies being the last resort but also the most effective [4, 8, 15–17]. Biological therapies work by suppressing the immune-mediated process that causes inflammation in most autoimmune disorders. There is a wide range of biological therapies available for treating moderate to severe psoriasis, depending on the pathway targeted by each agent [18].

2. Prevalence in population

Psoriasis is a common disease as such it has a global prevalence ranging between 0.91% and 8.5% [19, 20]. Some studies have shown that it affects around 1–3% of the population [21, 22]. Population-based studies indicate that psoriasis affects 2–3% of the UK population [23] approximately 1.7% of the Canadian population [6], 0.2–0.3% of Chinese/Taiwanese populations [24], and ≤1% of the population is affected in South Africa [25]. Age of onset is between the ages of 16–22 (early) and 57–60 (late) years [11, 25] and affects both genders equally [26, 27]. Significant differences in prevalence rates depended on whether the study population included children only or adults only, also whether individuals of all ages, as well as on the underlying age and sex structure of the whole population [20].

In a recent review commissioned as part of the World Health Organization (WHO) Global report on psoriasis, it was estimated that the prevalence of psoriasis ranged from 0.51% to 11.43% in adults and from 0% to 1.37% in children [28]. Although the prevalence was significant in this study, results could be debatable as reviewed data was provided from only 20 countries out of 194 WHO member states.

In the United Kingdom (UK), a cohort study indicated a prevalence of psoriasis from 2.3% (2297 cases per 100,000) in 1999 to 2.8% (2815 per 100,000) in 2013 while adult psoriasis ranged from 1.3% in the UK (95% CI:1.21–1.39) 5 to 8.5% in Norway (95% CI: 8.03–8.97) 6 depending on gender and geographic region [20, 23]. Other studies conducted in the United States of America (USA) among adults reported age- and sex-adjusted annual incidence of psoriasis as 62.3/100,000 if the diagnosis was restricted to dermatologist-confirmed subjects [28]. In Italy, a 5-year observational study reported a higher incidence among the adult population of – 321 and 230 per 100,000, in the year 2001 and 2005, respectively [29].

Psoriasis is common in women and certain ethnic groups; however, it was practically absent in Africa until the HIV pandemic [30, 31]. Prevalence studies reported the psoriasis incidence as 10.26 in Algeria, 15.04 in Morocco, and 13.26 in Tunisia per 1000 adults, and the study results were calculated based on a 2-week screening study via medical consultation [32]. Estimates in the Republic of Tanzania were the lowest at 0.96% [28]. In a survey of dermatology out-patients, involving five academic hospitals in South Africa (SA), Johannesburg, it was observed that there has been an increase in dermatological conditions, with psoriasis being the most common (9.6%) among Indian patients. The increase in dermatological conditions was associated with the HIV pandemic as it was first diagnosed in 1982 in SA [31]. Another study, which included mainly indigent [33] non-Caucasian South Africans in Johannesburg, showed that cardiometabolic disease is highly associated with severe psoriasis, and also, an association existed between increasing obesity and psoriasis. However, the findings of this study were limited as they may not be generalizable to all South African patients as data was collected from public hospitals [19].

3. Clinical types of psoriasis

The diagnosis of psoriasis is primarily clinical, based on the presence of erythematous scaly patches, pustules, and plaques (**Figure 1**) [10], and differs depending on the psoriasis variant [2, 10]. These variants include plaque psoriasis,

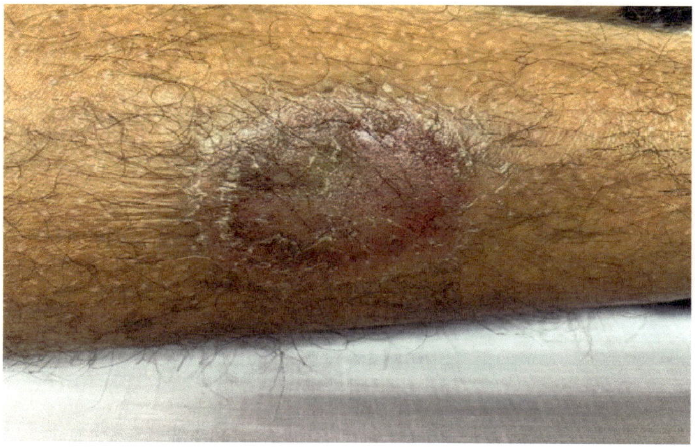

Figure 1.
Clinical features of psoriasis. Source: Image courtesy of Prof Dlova, Nelson Mandela Medical School, University of KwaZulu-Natal.

flexural, guttate psoriasis, erythrodermic psoriasis, and pustular psoriasis [6, 15]. Due to psoriasis being a disease of systemic inflammation, it is associated with multiple comorbidities such as psoriatic arthritis, cardiovascular disease, metabolic syndrome, obesity, hypertension, diabetes dyslipidemia, and depression [2, 3].

3.1 Plaque psoriasis

Plaque psoriasis also known as psoriasis vulgaris [5] is the most common variant presenting 80–90% of all manifestations of psoriasis. It occurs anywhere on the body (**Figure 2a** and **b**), commonly on extensor surfaces of the arms, legs, scalp buttocks, and trunk [10], but may also affect skin folding areas, palms, soles, and nails [2]. It is usually characterized by well-defined oval or round plaques which differ in size and often join together [10]. The pathogenesis of plaque psoriasis involves a feed-forward mechanism of inflammation predominantly including the T-helper cell type 17 (T_H17) pathway [2]. The affected areas are typically well-demarcated and systemic [2]. According to the Koebner phenomenon, stressful physiological, and psychological events and external factors are associated with the development of new lesions on sites of trauma, such as cuts, scratching, or pressure [2, 10]. Bleeding can occur when the dry scales are picked and lifted from the plaque. This is due to the skin under the scales being thin, making it more prone to damage [2].

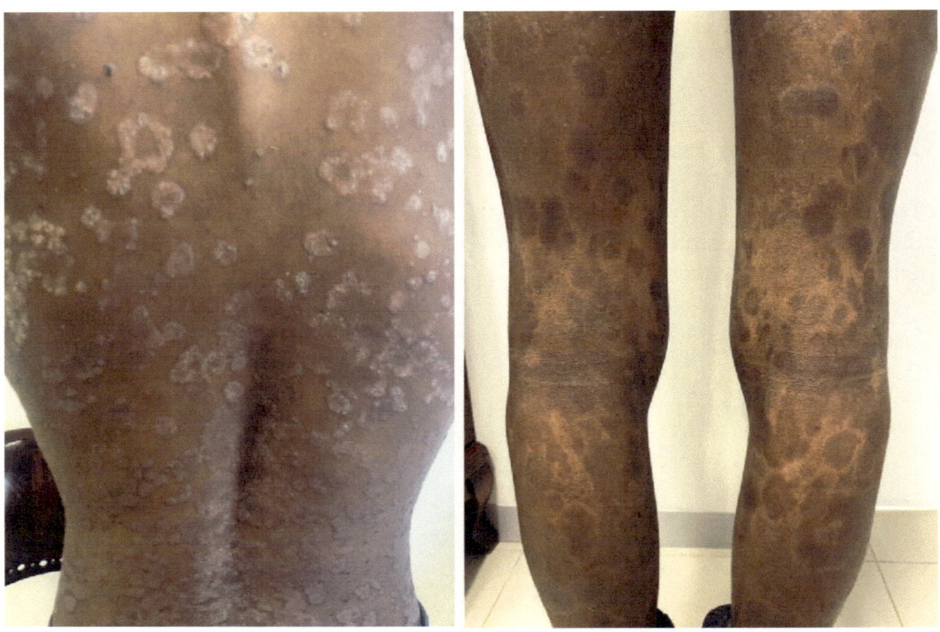

a) b)

Figure 2.
Chronic plaque-type psoriasis with erythematous well-demarcated plaques covered with silvery scales. (a) Full back involvement. (b) Legs involvement. Source: Image courtesy of Prof Dlova, Nelson Mandela Medical School, University of KwaZulu-Natal.

3.2 Flexural psoriasis

Inverse psoriasis, also called flexural psoriasis [5], is less scaly than plaque psoriasis. It is characterized by slightly erosive erythematous patches occurring in the intertriginous locations of the flexor surfaces and perineal area, such as the axillary, inguinal, and intergluteal folds (**Figure 3**) [5].

3.3 Guttate psoriasis

Guttate psoriasis (**Figure 4**) is characterized by multiple 3–5 mm confetti-like scaly pink patches [2] and causes an acute systemic eruption of papules or plaques mainly on the trunk and limbs [15]. Guttate psoriasis usually affects children and adolescents [5]. It makes up 2% of psoriasis cases, and approximately 66% of new-onset guttate psoriasis are led by an upper respiratory tract infection such as streptococcal infection [2]. In some cases, these resolve naturally within weeks to months, however, can also become chronic [2], and may later develop into plaque psoriasis [15].

3.4 Erythrodermic psoriasis

Erythrodermic psoriasis (**Figure 5**) is characterized by widespread generalized erythema and inflammation covering 90% of the total body surface [5]. Although it only occurs in 2–3% of psoriasis cases, it requires emergency treatment due to it being associated with systemic symptoms [10] and can be life-threatening due to complications such as hypothermia, risk of infection, acute kidney injury, and cardiac failure [15]. Development may be slow from long-standing psoriasis or may appear abruptly in patients who present with mild psoriasis [10].

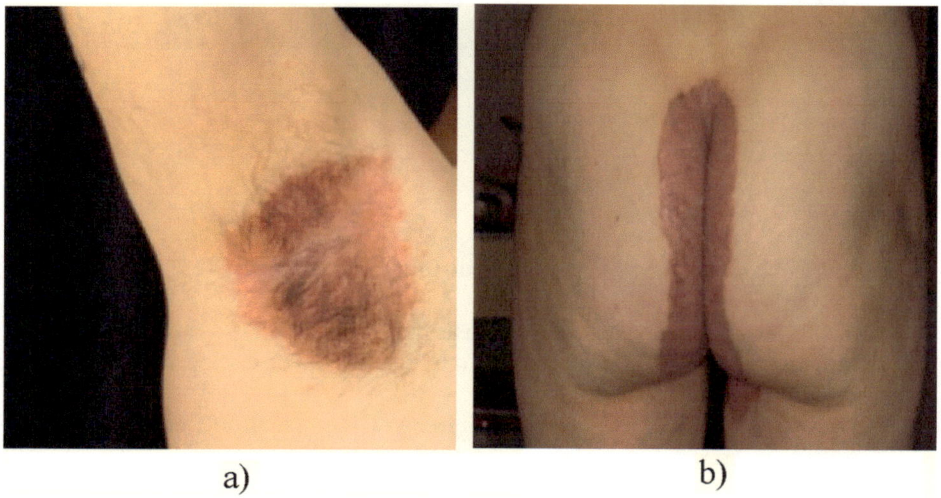

Figure 3.
Clinical involvement of the skin folds [5]. (a) Axillary fold involvement. (b) Intergluteal involvement.

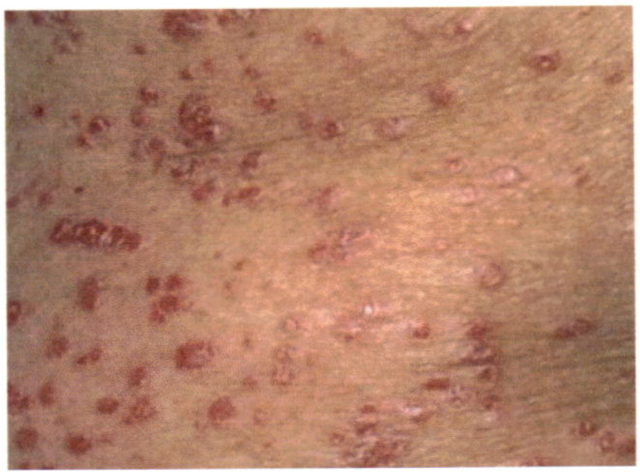

Figure 4.
Clinical manifestation of guttate psoriasis [5].

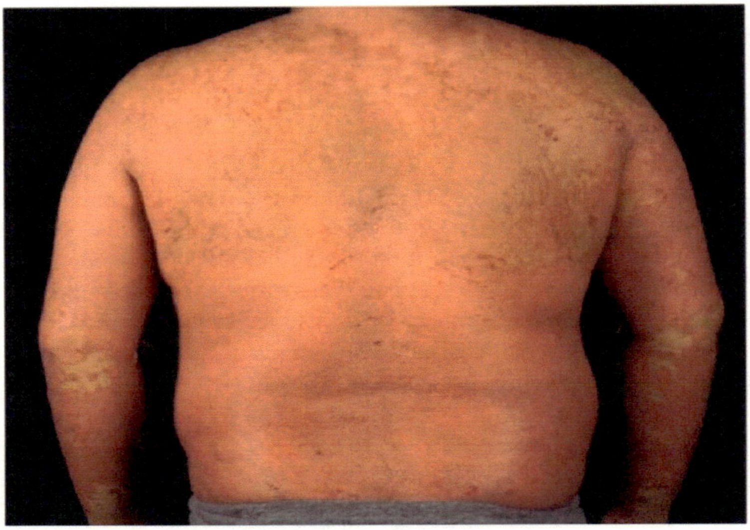

Figure 5.
Clinical manifestation of erythrodermic psoriasis [5].

3.5 Pustular psoriasis

Pustular psoriasis is characterized by multiple sterile pustules [15]. It can be localized or generalized (**Figure 6**).

Localized phenotypes of pustular psoriasis have been described as psoriasis pustulosa palmo-plantaris (PPP) and acrodermatitis continua of Hallopeau (ACH) which both affect the hands and feet (**Figure 7**).

PPP is limited to the palms and soles, whereas ACH presents at the fingertips and toe tips and affects the nail apparatus [5]. Localized pustular psoriasis can negatively impact day-to-day activities [15]. Generalized pustular psoriasis (GPP) can present acutely and rapidly progress with a widespread eruption of superficial pustules. It is often accompanied by systemic symptoms and can be life-threatening [5, 15]. Various treatment types are available to treat mild to severe psoriasis.

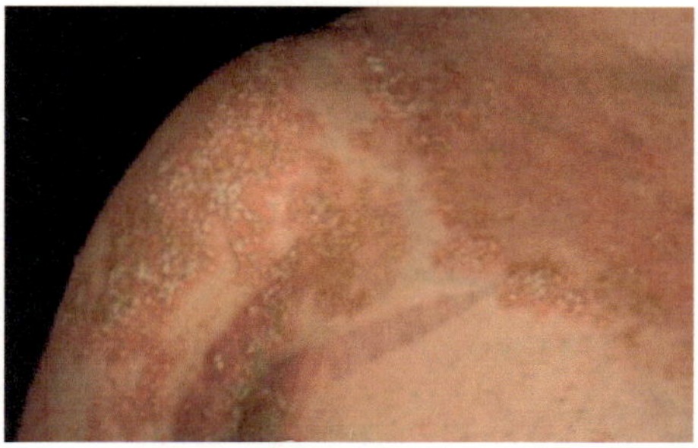

Figure 6.
Clinical manifestation of generalized pustular psoriasis [5].

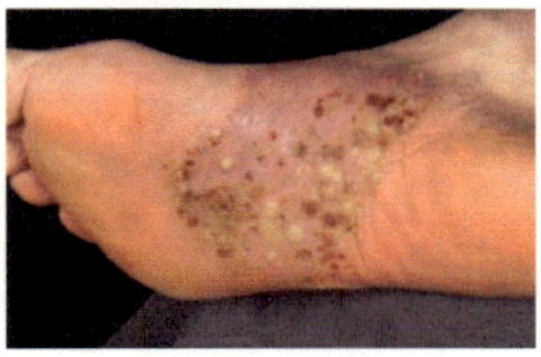

Figure 7.
Clinical manifestation of pustular psoriasis localized to the soles of the feet [5].

3.6 Psoriatic arthritis (PsA)

It is estimated that about 14–40% of people who suffer from psoriasis develop PsA [34–37]. It is estimated that 15% of those suffering from psoriasis have undetected PsA [38]. PsA is characterized by involvement of the metacarpophalangeal and interphalangeal joints of the hands and feet, as well as the ankles and knees [38]. There can also be extra-articular involvement, such as eye and/or bowel involvement, and occasionally involvement of the sacroiliac joints and/or the spinal cord [10]. Other distinguishing features of PsA include the absence of rheumatoid factor and anti-cyclic citrullinated peptide (CCP) antibodies [39]. Through ultrasonography and magnetic resonance imaging, it has been discovered that the enthesis might be the first site of inflammation in PsA [40]. When compared to rheumatoid arthritis (RA), PsA is distinguished by synovium inflammation which is characterized by more intense hypervascularity and infiltration of polymorphonuclear leukocytes [39, 40]. Moreover, PsA is frequently associated with HLA-B27 in patients who have axial involvement [41]. These findings suggest that angiogenesis plays a central role in the early events in PsA.

Clinically (**Figure 8**), PsA manifests with oligoarticular or polyarticular dactylitis and enthesitis, which the polyarticular variety is commonly linked with nail involvement [42]. Psoriatic nail involvement has been associated with joint involvement, and nail manifestations can occur in as many as 80% of patients who suffer from PsA [43]. The clinical appearance of nail psoriasis is determined by the structure impacted by the inflammatory process. Pitting, leukonychia, and onychodystrophy are symptoms of nail matrix involvement, whereas oil-drop discoloration, splinter hemorrhages, and onychodystrophy are symptoms of nail bed inflammation [43–45].

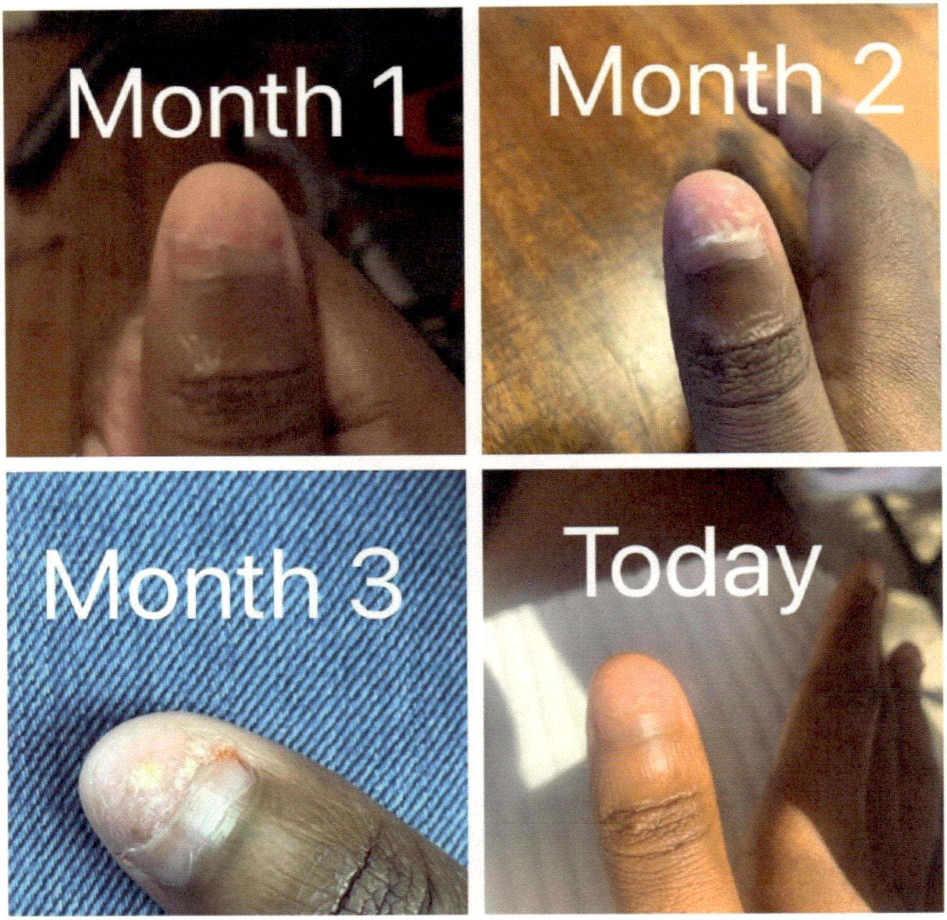

Figure 8.
Psoriatic arthritis with nail involvement. Source: Image courtesy of Prof Dlova, Nelson Mandela Medical School, University of KwaZulu-Natal.

4. Association of psoriasis to different organ systems

Although psoriasis affects the skin, being a metabolic syndrome it may also affect the joints and has been associated with numerous diseases since inflammation is not limited to the skin but can affect different organ systems as well [5]. These comorbidities include psoriatic arthritis, cardiovascular disease, Crohn's disease, mild liver disease, chronic kidney disease, end-stage kidney disease, obesity, hypertension, diabetes, and dyslipidemia [3, 46–50]. Large studies have shown that a higher occurrence of patients with cardiovascular disease and diabetes correlates with the severity of psoriasis [51–53].

Obesity is more prevalent and common in people who suffer from psoriasis compared to the general population [54]. While the exact mechanism underlying the link between psoriasis and obesity is unknown, a number of studies of basic as well as translational research indicate that adipocytes and inflammatory-type macrophages may play a role in both disease processes [54]. The adipose tissue is a living endocrine organ that regulates lipid and glucose metabolism, inflammation and coagulation, and insulin-mediated processes [55, 56]. Macrophages are the primary immune cell type responsible for adipose tissue inflammation. Adipose tissue-activated macrophages stimulate adipocytes to secrete inflammatory mediators that promote and sustain an inflammatory state in obesity. Adipose tissue, in particular visceral adipose tissue, secretes bioactive products known as adipocytokines or adipokines. The function of adipokines and their downstream effects are thought to play a role in the coexistence of psoriasis and obesity [6, 55–58].

Due to the notably weight gain, people who suffer from psoriasis may not be motivated to participate in physical activity due to the appearance of their skin as well weight gain which they may be embarrassed about. Considered together, the various elements that contribute to psoriasis as a systemic illness can have a substantial impact on patient's quality of life and disease burden. The high disease burden is assumed to be due to the disease's symptoms, which include discomfort, pruritus, and bleeding, in addition to the previously mentioned related conditions.

5. Treatment interventions

Psoriasis often requires long-term therapy [5], which can control the signs and symptoms [59]. There are various treatment options ranging from mild, to moderate to severe [2], and the choice of therapy is determined by the severity of the psoriasis, comorbidities, and access to health care [5]. First-line treatment for mild psoriasis includes topical agents such as vitamin D analogues and corticosteroids. Phototherapy such as narrowband ultraviolet B radiation (NB-UVB), psoralen with ultraviolet A radiation (PUVA), and conventional systemic agents (methotrexate, ciclosporin, and acitretin) are used as second-line therapy [15] for moderate to severe psoriasis [2]. Additional treatments include targeted biologics (tumor necrosis factor (TNF), interleukin (IL)-17, and IL-23 inhibitors), as well as oral molecule inhibitors (dimethyl fumarate and a premilast) [15].

5.1 Vitamin D analogues

Vitamin D analogues are a first-line topical agent for treating plaque psoriasis and scalp psoriasis [6]. Vitamin D analogues such as calcipotriol bind to vitamin D receptors on T-cells and to vitamin D receptors on keratinocytes. This causes a blockage of keratinocyte proliferation and increases keratinocyte differentiation [2]. The effectiveness of topical agents is modest when used on its own [2]; however, it can be increased with occlusion or combination therapy with systemic agents [15]. Randomized trials have shown that vitamin D is safe and effective for patients with mild psoriasis; however, it is not inferior to most corticosteroids [4, 60].

5.2 Corticosteroids

Topical corticosteroid therapy is used to treat patients with mild or localized psoriasis. Corticosteroids are considered the cornerstone of topical treatments and are often well tolerated when used as prescribed and effective at appropriate strengths for patients [2, 6]. Their method of operation is to exert anti-inflammatory, antiproliferative, and local vasoconstriction effects through the downregulation of genes coding proinflammatory cytokines [2].

5.3 Phototherapy

Phototherapy such as psoralen plus UVA (PUVA), broadband UVB, and narrowband UVB (NB-UVB) treats moderate to severe psoriasis, especially those that are unresponsive to topical treatment agents [6]. Treatment using narrowband UV-B is preferred over broadband UV-B due to it being more effective. The narrowband UV-B is also preferred over PUVA [2] due to the risks of skin cancer with cumulative doses of PUVA [15].

UV-B: UV-B therapy consists of broadband (290–320 nm) and narrowband (311 nm) bandwidths which are both able to treat plaque psoriasis [2]. The treatment can be administered in a clinic office or at home usually three times per week. After 2–3 months, the treatment frequency can be decreased to twice a week to maintain the treatment results. Adverse effects of UV-B phototherapy include erythema, pruritus, blistering, photoaging, and photo-carcinogenesis [2].

Although there is no evidence that NB-UVB increases the risk of skin cancer [6], it is most commonly used due to its greater effectiveness and decreased adverse effects [2]. NB-UVB treatment can be given to almost any patient, including children and pregnant women [6]. A combination of systemic retinoids may also increase the effectiveness and reduce potential carcinogenic adverse effects of NB-UVB [2].

5.4 PUVA

Psoralen plus UVA involves a combination treatment consisting of a psoralen such as methoxalen which is either administered orally or topically before being exposed to long-wave UV-A (320–400 nm) irradiation [2]. Psoralens cause the skin to become temporarily sensitive to UVA and interject into DNA to suppress DNA synthesis [2]. PUVA treatment can initially be administered two to three times per week. Once the psoriasis is almost clear, or clear, the frequency is then decreased. Adverse effects include gastrointestinal upset, burning, pruritus, hypertrichosis, and photoaging. The effectiveness of PUVA is superior to UV-B; however, it is no longer the preferred treatment due to the risks of skin malignancies with long-term use [2, 15]. The use of phototherapy for moderate to severe psoriasis has decreased since the introduction of biologics [2].

5.5 Systemic agents

- *Methotrexate*—Methotrexate is a folate derivative that inhibits several enzymes responsible for nucleotide synthesis that leads to the suppression of inflammation and prevention of cell division [15]. Potential complications include nausea, vomiting, diarrhea, fatigue pneumonitis, hepatitis, liver fibrosis, and teratogenicity [6, 15]. Its most serious adverse effects include bone marrow suppression [6]. Due to its toxic adverse effect, it is used to treat moderately severe to severe psoriasis if first-line treatments have failed, as well as psoriatic arthritis [6]. Methotrexate is also contraindicated in pregnancy [15].

- *Cyclosporine* is a calcineurin inhibitor [61] used in the treatment of moderate to severe psoriasis [6]. Cyclosporine works rapidly to suppress the immune system and slows down the growth of certain immune cells [15]. Adverse effects include nephrotoxicity, hepatoxicity, hypertension, increased risk of infection, lymphoma, tremors, hyperplasia, drug interactions, and malignancies [6, 61]

- *Acitretin* is a synthetic oral retinoid used in the treatment of moderate to severe psoriasis [5]. It normalizes keratinocyte proliferation and differentiation [15]. Its function as an adjunctive therapy has been reported to enhance efficacy, lower doses, and reduce the occurrence of side effects [6]. The side effects of Acitretin include hair loss, dry skin, high cholesterol, and liver damage. Acitretin is also contraindicated in pregnancy [15].

5.6 Biologics

Biologic therapy is one of the most significant therapeutic advancements in dermatology for the treatment of psoriasis [2] and has been developed as a highly potent treatment for patients who are unresponsive to traditional systemic treatments or are not tolerated due to adverse effects or comorbidities [6]. These drugs are monoclonal antibodies or soluble receptors [15] which target specific parts of the immune system that overact in psoriasis. They are medicines made from living cells that are genetically changed in a laboratory to make certain proteins. Biologics are designed to block only the parts of the immune system that are responsible for the overgrowth of skin cells [62] and have a dramatic effect on the outcome of moderate to severe psoriasis [15]. Approved biologic therapies include TNF (adalimumab, etanercept, infliximab, and certolizumab), IL-17 (ixekizumab and secukinumab), IL-17 receptor inhibitors (brodalumab) and IL-12/23 rizankizumab, guselkumab, and tildrakizumab [15]. Biologic therapies can be administered as a shot or an infusion through an IV drip [62].

TNF inhibitors—Tumor necrosis factor (TNF) is considered the oldest approved biologic treatment for psoriasis [63]. TNF therapists include adalimumab, etanercept, infliximab, and certolizumab. While all blocks of TNF in vivo, they differ in structure and mechanism of action [63]. These biologics decrease the downstream inflammatory cascade central to the psoriasis pathogenesis. Among the TNF-a inhibitors for psoriasis, infliximab has the highest efficacy, followed by certolizumab and adalimumab and then etanercept being the least effective [2]. The most common adverse effects are nasopharyngitis, upper respiratory tract infection, and injection site reactions [2].

Interleukin-12/23 (IL-12/23) targets a type of cytokine called IL-23 which are a class of proteins that help transmit signals from one cell to another. The role of IL-23 signals pathways that trigger inflammation. The IL-23 inhibitors block this action which helps limit the inflammation that causes psoriasis symptoms [2]. Types of IL-23 inhibitors include Guselkumab, Rizankizumab, and Tildrakizumab. IL-23 inhibitors cause fewer side effects, and adverse effects are very rare. Adverse effects include upper respiratory infections, certain fungal infections, herpes simplex infections, and infectious diarrhea [64].

Interleukin-17 (IL-17) is a class of biological therapy that targets either the IL-17 ligand or its receptors. They have a rapid onset of action, robust response, and great sustainability in treating plaque psoriasis. There are three types of monoclonal antibodies of IL-17 inhibitors which [5] include ixekizumab, secukinumab, and brodalumab. IL-17 inhibitors have an acceptable safety profile with no increased risks of serious infections or malignancies [2]. The main adverse effects are candidiasis, neutropenia, inflammatory bowel disease and depression, and the risk of suicide in brodalumab [61].

6. Effects of psoriasis on quality of life

The World Health Organization (WHO) defines quality of life (QoL) as an individual's perception of their position in life, concerning their goals, expectations, standards, and concerns, in the context of the culture and value system in which they live [65]. Being a visible skin disorder, psoriasis has a significant impact on the quality of life. It is widely accepted today and has been known since ancient times in Ayurveda that there is an association between the skin and the mind [66]. As such psoriasis causes stress and has an impact on self-image, psoriasis can trigger processes that lower self-esteem and can contribute to feelings like anxiety, sadness, or even depression [67, 68]. Reciprocally, psoriasis is evoked by stress [59, 66, 69, 70].

Psoriasis can cause physical distress, pain, and itching, which can negatively impact a patient's daily activities and well-being [71]. Psoriasis patients may also encounter psychological and social challenges, such as stigmatization, humiliation, and social inhibition [60]. Additionally, smoking and alcohol abuse are more prevalent perhaps as a consequence or as a coping mechanism [60, 70]. Children and adolescents also experience a substantial impact on the quality of life as their physical, psychosocial, and emotional health gets affected [72, 73]. The disease symptoms such as societal stigmatization, appearance-related social anxiety, impairment of professional activities as well as the lack of a cure-all have a negative impact on the perceptions of those who suffer from psoriasis [68, 74].

Its impact on QoL largely depends on the severity and type. For example, palmoplantar psoriasis, i.e., an affliction of the palms of the hands and soles of the feet, has been linked to a greater decline in health-related quality of life compared with moderate-to-severe plaque psoriasis [75]. Patients with palmoplantar psoriasis were more likely to report moderate impairments in quality of life, mobility, self-care, and routine activities [37]. Gånemo et al., for example, discovered that joint complaints and pruritus substantially diminish the QoL of patients [73].

Contrary to intuition, the impact on QoL does not necessarily correlate to the severity of psoriasis. However, the subjective experience of psoriasis is a stronger predictor of QoL than severity [72]. The psychological burden of psoriasis can range from mild reductions in quality of life to suicidal thoughts [76]. Psoriasis can also adversely affect relationships and environmental aspects of QoL [77]. In addition, psoriasis can have economic consequences too. The economic impact of psoriasis increases as disease severity worsens, resulting in greater psychosocial morbidity [78] decreased work productivity, higher healthcare costs, and diminished QoL [40].

6.1 Measuring QoL in psoriasis

Various instruments and questionnaires can be used to evaluate the QoL for psoriasis patients. The most common is the Dermatology Life Quality Index (DLQI). DLQI is a self-administered questionnaire that assesses the impact of skin diseases on various aspects of a patient's life [75] such as effects on daily activities, work or school performance, intimate relationships, and emotional well-being [55, 56]. Higher DLQI scores indicate a larger decline in QoL. Likewise, another clinical assessment tool questionnaire for psoriasis, the Psoriasis Area and Severity Index (PASI) does not appropriately measure the impact that the condition has on patients' lives but rather offers only an index of clinical severity based on clinical appearance [1].

In dermatology, the perception of quality of life is regarded as a critical metric. In this sense, quality of life assessment has evolved into an indicator used to guide healthcare practices and aid in the development of public policy strategies [68, 79]. Public health policies are needed to increase the general population's knowledge and awareness of psoriasis. This approach may help to explain the impact of psoriasis on a person's life, reducing prejudice and facilitating social inclusion [79, 80].

The Children's Dermatology Life Quality Index (CDLQI) and the Infant's Dermatitis Quality of Life Index (IDQOL) are additional questionnaires that evaluate the effect of psoriasis on the QoL of children and adolescents [73]. These instruments accommodate the unique difficulties and experiences of younger psoriasis patients. There is currently a need to improve the quality of life measures for psoriasis patients to determine issues that are significant to them, such as disease prejudice, stigma, and social injustices [68]. It has also been discovered that social support plays a role in adjusting to life with psoriasis [81]. There is a correlation between higher levels of social support and improved QoL and lower levels of depression, and therefore, a form of tangible support is crucial for enhancing acceptance of life with psoriasis [72, 81].

6.2 Effective treatments known to improve QoL in psoriasis patients

Both systemic and topical therapies are effective treatments for psoriasis patients who want to enhance their QoL. Systemic therapies, such as biologic agents (e.g., TNF inhibitors and IL-17 inhibitors) and non-biologic systemic agents (e.g., methotrexate and cyclosporine), have demonstrated considerable efficacy in reducing psoriasis symptoms and enhancing QoL [82]. These treatments target the underlying immune dysregulation associated with psoriasis and can result in long-term remission or marked improvement of symptoms [42]. Topical therapies for localized psoriasis, such as corticosteroids, vitamin D analogues, and calcineurin inhibitors, can provide symptomatic relief and enhance QoL [82] which are generally well-tolerated and can be combined with systemic therapies for increased efficacy [42].

Psychosocial interventions such as cognitive-behavioral therapy (CBT) can help patients manage the emotional and social effects of psoriasis and improve their overall health [83]. Individuals with psoriasis can benefit from patient education, support groups, and counseling as additional resources and support. Importantly, the choice of therapy should be individualized based on disease severity, comorbidities, patient preferences, and treatment objectives [82]. To ensure optimal control over symptoms and minimize the impact on QoL, regular monitoring and adjustment of treatment regimens are required.

6.3 What patients can do to reduce its effects

Several evidence-based strategies can be employed to mitigate the impact on QoL. These strategies seek to alleviate the physical symptoms of psoriasis, mitigate its psychological effects, and improve overall health. Establishing treatment objectives for psoriasis is of paramount importance for enhancing patient care and reducing the problem of undertreatment [84]. The severity of the disease should determine the treatment objectives, which may include reducing the affected body surface area and minimizing the impact on QoL [84]. Implementing this holistic treatment approach in daily psoriasis management can help guide treatment decisions and ensure better outcomes.

Systemic therapy may be required for moderate to severe psoriasis. Specific objectives can be established for the induction and maintenance phases of treatment [33]. Its selection should, once again, be individualized for each patient [85]. To ensure optimal control of symptoms and minimize the impact on QoL, regular monitoring and adjustment of treatment regimens are essential [33].

The psychosocial burden of psoriasis should not be disregarded. It is necessary to include psychosocial morbidity measures when evaluating psoriasis severity and treatment efficacy [86]. Psychosocial support and counseling can help patients manage the emotional and social effects of psoriasis [87]. Mediation cognitive-behavioral therapy (MCBT) has been demonstrated to be effective in this regard [46]. The MCBT technique helps to teach patients to focus their attention and maintain positive thinking. It is believed that patients practicing meditation can detach from the negative emotions associated with psoriasis [88].

People living with chronic psoriasis are encouraged to adhere to their treatment plan, for example, use their medication as prescribed. Non-adherence to medication often results in missed opportunities to optimize the efficacy of a treatment, and dermatologists should embrace a nonjudgmental approach and accept non-adherence as the norm [89]. Studies have revealed that non-adherence is due to psychological distress from a patient's inability to manage his or her condition resulting in reduced motivation or they get worried about the treatment side effects [90].

Lifestyle changes should be an important consideration. The World Health Organization identifies insufficient physical activity as a key risk factor for cardiovascular diseases, cancer, and diabetes [91]. Patients with moderate to severe psoriasis are especially vulnerable to suboptimal lifestyles because they have an elevated risk of both cardiovascular and metabolic disease [91]. Consequently, a suboptimal lifestyle is particularly dangerous and has a negative impact on psoriasis itself. Lifestyle improvement for patients with psoriasis may involve numerous areas of improvement such as diet, smoking, alcohol, and relaxation techniques. However, physical activity should be highly encouraged given the apparent positive influence on psoriasis itself alongside the potential cardiovascular and metabolic comorbidities associated with psoriasis [91].

Relaxation therapies should form part of the treatment regimen. Holistic treatments used in the management of psoriasis include aromatherapy, massage, spa therapies, mud baths, and flotation tanks. Aromatherapy uses therapeutic blends of oils to allow healing and relaxation and to lift a patient's mood [1, 92]. Manipulative techniques are beneficial as they help with pain reduction and increase joint mobility in the case of psoriatic arthritis; massage is the most popular technique used [93].

Mud applications are usually in the form of packs and baths, with the head not being immersed. The most common indicated treatments are moor mud baths which incorporate dead sea mud [94]. The mud bath provides a notable increase in magnesium and bromine in the skin, both of these compounds might play a vital role in psoriatic skin [94–96]. While the mud bath is not accepted as a well-established treatment modality due to a lack of clinical trials, thermal balneotherapy is used throughout the world in psoriatic therapy owing to its ability to offer natural, multifactorial, complementary, and nontoxic alternative treatments [95, 96]. The most important attribute of the therapy for psoriatic patients is safety; many of them accept the possibility of using safe natural treatments with enthusiasm despite their variable efficacy [1].

The skin barrier function in psoriatic skin is compromised, as such, hydration therapy becomes a key factor. Hydrating treatments offered in a skin care clinic or a health spa such as balneotherapy using the dead sea mud could help enhance the cutaneous barrier function as well as address hydration of the stratum corneum [1, 94]. The use of products with natural ingredients such as *Aloe vera* could help restore the disturbed skin's barrier function as they have hydrating properties [1, 97].

7. Psychosocial management of psoriasis

Visible psoriatic lesions on exposed body parts can elicit feelings of anxiety, disgust, aversion, and even intolerance [81, 98]. Furthermore, some people who are unfamiliar or with limited knowledge of psoriasis believe that the disease is contagious, which may further contribute to the social isolation of people with psoriasis [86, 98]. People who suffer from psoriasis are often in denial and suffer from a great deal of stigmatization [98]. There are two types of stigma: social stigma (social exclusion and unfair discriminatory treatment) and self-stigma (low self-esteem with feelings of shame and hopelessness as a result of the disease) [99–101]. According to Goffman's theory, stigmatized people are rejected as a result of having a deeply discredited attribute in their society [102].

Both social and self-stigmatization can occur independently, but they can also coexist [98, 100]. People who have psoriasis are vulnerable to comments and remarks about their disease, which can lead to social withdrawal, depression, and even suicide attempts [103]. Additionally, the internalization of illness-related stigma can lead to feelings of guilt, and the fear of being judged by others can jeopardize one's emotional state and even lead to mental illness [104]. Due to stigmatization, people with psoriasis often experience loneliness in addition to decreased quality of life, which further impairs their social functioning [98, 100]. Loneliness is caused by physical and mental illnesses, as well as psychological disturbances such as low self-esteem, inability to establish social contacts, and stigmatization [103, 104].

A recent scholarly review by Nguyen et al. on the psychosocial impact of acne, vitiligo, and psoriasis suggests that all these conditions have a negative psychosocial impact on the affected individual in that conditions result in increased levels of anxiety and depression among patients [80]. Another similar study conducted in Croatia found that while depression and anxiety were prevalent among patients affected by psoriasis, gender differences existed concerning the extent of anxiety and depressive symptoms [105]. Another study conducted to investigate the impact of psoriasis on quality of life and explore the determinant factors found that there is a close relationship between stress and the disease. This perpetuates a vicious cycle, which may explain the cause of the disease in certain instances and others may exacerbate the negative symptoms leading to poor treatment and a deteriorated health state [106].

Strober et al. [107] reported that moderate to severe psoriasis as manifested by poor patient outcomes was attributed to a longer stay away from work which subsequently has occupational and financial implications for the individual diagnosed with the condition. Similarly, other studies on patient outcomes related to psoriasis have also reported that the condition has physically and mentally debilitating effects on one's life, thus necessitating psychological and educational interventions [108]. Earlier studies conducted on the quality of life and work productivity impairment among psoriasis patients have also revealed that patients who experience arthritic symptoms associated with the disease suffer significant impairments related to the quality of life and occupational productivity [109].

Similar studies conducted among children and adolescents also suggest that psoriasis has a negative impact on quality of life. There is evidence to suggest that the prevalence of psoriasis among children and adolescents may perpetuate learning difficulties and disturbances in school. The condition may also lead to long-term sequel of mental health disorders among children with consequences to family life [83]. The families affected by the individual diagnosed with psoriasis could also face financial burdens associated with the disease. Since stigma is also a consequence faced by the individual, associative stigma is also faced by families who have their family members diagnosed with the condition.

Based on current empirical evidence, there is consensus among authors that the condition greatly affects the quality of life as it has a profoundly negative impact on the affected individuals' self-image, self-esteem, and overall sense of personal well-being [110, 111]. Studies conducted on the impact of the diagnosis of psoriasis on the individual have suggested that the condition affects all aspects of life including psychological, physical, social, sexual, and occupational components [112, 113].

Due to the multiple effects of the condition, a strictly biomedical approach to managing the condition may result in unmet health needs of individuals affected by the condition. Empirical evidence alludes to the multiplicity of effects that the condition has which extends beyond the individual to include family and other individuals of influence. In addition to the adoption of standardized medical interventions encompassing diagnostics, treatment, and related follow-up procedures, the psychosocial management plan thus becomes an integral part of facilitating the holistic management of the patient. This psychosocial management approach must be tailored to the individual's needs and should be cognizant of various socio-demographic factors that may affect the health and health-seeking behaviors of the patient diagnosed with psoriasis.

The health interventions that should form part of the psychosocial approach to managing these clients are thus formulated with the health worker adopting a holistic and comprehensive lens of enquiry to understand the challenges and needs faced by individuals diagnosed with psoriasis. In this regard, drawing on the discipline of health promotion, social sciences, and behavioral sciences becomes necessary if effective interventions are to be designed and offered to patients. Psychological intervention programs should consider patients' opinions and attitudes toward their illness, their level of self-acceptance, and the emotions associated with the disease, and also, non-pharmacological interventions such as biofeedback, relaxation training, and cognitive behavioral therapy may improve patients' quality of life [98].

The socio-ecological model for understanding the health needs and challenges of people with varying health conditions is an example of a theoretical lens of enquiry that may be adopted by health workers in the enquiry process [114]. It may help to frame the specific areas of intervention that may be directed at the individual level and population levels especially if a large-scale public health intervention is to be designed for a specific community or society of individuals that may be affected by psoriasis.

At the individual level, health workers in these instances are to be empathic toward patients, provide relevant counseling advice as needed, and be on the alert for anxiety and depressive symptoms so that relevant psychotherapy and intervention may be provided. The skin specialist (dermatologist) and healthcare provider managing the patient diagnosed with psoriasis must be equipped with the necessary knowledge and skills to manage the condition from a holistic perspective. The healthcare provider must be able to address queries and concerns that the patient may have about the nature of the condition and the side effects of treatment. Before the treatment intervention is chosen, patients must be allowed to be an integral part of decision-making about the treatment process, so that informed decisions are taken.

In this regard, healthcare workers are to ensure that patients have information about various treatment options with specific discussion about the risk-benefit ratio concerning physical well-being and overall health. The patient should also be made aware of any cost implications related to the treatment process and the anticipated outcomes concerning the management of the condition. Through the provision of comprehensive information, the patient is empowered to exercise their right to autonomy which is critical in instances of debilitating conditions as one's self-worth is often compromised in the process. Allowing patients an opportunity to ask questions, clarify misconceptions, and empower them to make their own decisions could be an effective means of considering a patient's sense of self-worth and esteem which are often compromised in such conditions.

Being able to develop screening mechanisms to assess the extent to which psoriasis has affected quality of life is also an important factor and is one of the first steps to ensuring that patients are holistically managed in terms of their psychosocial needs. The development of validated screening tools for patient function concerning physical, mental, emotional, occupation, and spiritual well-being. These screening tools could also be effective in terms of problem identification so that relevant supportive measures may be instituted. In the cases of mental and emotional disturbances related to the condition, relevant interventions in the form of counseling and supportive rehabilitative, promotive, and curative therapy using a combination of approaches through biomedicine, cognitive behavioral therapy, and alternative practices have been proven to be effective at managing the psychological stresses that may be associated with the condition [98].

Another key aspect of psychosocial management is the assessment and prevention of complications associated with physical impairments that are related to psoriasis. In this regard, prevention may be facilitated through education regarding various approaches to prevent situations that may lead to immobility and related complications. Moreover, in instances of side effects such as arthritis, management also entails referral to other physical therapists who may further educate or institute measures to maximize mobility.

In instances where children and adolescents are affected by psoriasis, an integral part of psychosocial management also entails managing the family of the child or adolescent. In such instances, the family is often overwhelmed by the diagnosis due to the complications associated with the disease. Moreover, the financial implications of treatment have a strain on individual family members and the family unit. Provision of counseling to the family as a unit thus also becomes important so that they are empowered on how to deal with the condition. Moreover, counseling may also help them to come to terms with the diagnosis and understand the role that they have to play in the treatment process. The family of a child, adolescent, or even adult diagnosed with psoriasis may also be at risk for associative stigma by their relation to someone diagnosed with psoriasis. Research on stigma by association as reported in other non-communicable diseases has suggested that associative stigma is a determinant for health-seeking behavior both from the part of the family and the individual affected by the condition [98–100]. Assisting families through the provision of mental support and counseling against stigma thus becomes important for instituting sustained treatment options.

In low- to middle-income settings with a high burden of communicable and non-communicable diseases, adopting differentiated models of care is effective at managing health conditions [115]. The adoption of a differentiated approach to care and management of psoriasis within a low- to middle-income context has important public health implications within the context of multi-morbidity. This is because the differentiated approach allows for patient self-management within the context of an in-depth understanding of multiple determinants affecting their health and access to care. Through a differentiated approach, patient-centered care is provided whilst upholding the universal principles of primary health care.

8. Conclusions

Psoriasis is linked to a slew of comorbidities, particularly cardiovascular diseases, which are the leading cause of death worldwide. Due to its physical discomfort, pain, irritation, and numerous psychological and social challenges, psoriasis has a significant impact on the QoL. Its impact is dependent on the type and its severity with palmoplantar psoriasis and joint complaints causing the greatest impairment on QoL.

Topical therapies remain the cornerstone for treating mild psoriasis, whereas phototherapy, systemic, and biologic therapy are used to treat moderate to severe psoriasis; however, there are various adverse effects associated with each treatment option and depending on the severity of psoriasis determines the treatment option used and is carefully evaluated. The subjective experience of disease should be a more important determinant of overall QoL than objective severity measurements.

To resolve the complex effects of psoriasis, a comprehensive and holistic strategy is required. Diet, non-smoking, no consumption of alcohol, and relaxation techniques can all help patients with psoriasis improve their lifestyle. However, given the apparent positive influence on psoriasis itself, as well as the potential cardiovascular and metabolic comorbidities associated with psoriasis, physical activity should be considered a starting point. Dermatologists ought to cease treating psoriasis as if it were a single skin condition rather than a complex condition requiring a discussion of lifestyle choices.

In addition to treating physical symptoms, the patient's psychological and emotional health should be highly considered. Increased stress has been demonstrated to have a negative impact on psoriasis. Alternative stress management therapies such as hydrating and spa therapies using dead sea mud and/or balneotherapy may be effective in stress management to improve overall well-being and QoL. Psychosocial support interventions should also be incorporated into a psoriasis management plan to help those who suffer from psoriasis cope with the stigmatization, thereby improving their quality of life.

Acknowledgements

We would like to acknowledge Professors, Ncoza Dlova and Knut Schäkel, for providing us with the photographs.

Conflict of interests

The authors declare no conflict of interest.

Psoriasis: Clinical Features and Its Impact on Quality of Life
DOI: http://dx.doi.org/10.5772/intechopen.1005098

Author details

Nomakhosi Mpofana[1*], Mokgadi Makgobole[1],
Celenkosini Thembelenkosini Nxumalo[2,3] and Pavitra Pillay[4]

1 Faculty of Health Sciences, Department of Somatology, Durban University of Technology, Durban, South Africa

2 Faculty of Health Sciences, Academic Development Unit, Durban University of Technology, Durban, South Africa

3 Discipline of Nursing, School of Nursing and Public Health, University of KwaZulu-Natal, South Africa

4 Faculty of Health Sciences, Department of Biomedical and Clinical Technology, Durban University of Technology, Durban, South Africa

*Address all correspondence to: nomakhosim@dut.ac.za

References

[1] Mpofana N, Maitland Griffiths CE, Dlova NC. The feasibility of an interdisciplinary approach on the management of psoriasis in South Africa. Alternative Therapies in Health & Medicine. 2022;**28**(2):58-64

[2] Armstrong AW, Read C. Pathophysiology, clinical presentation, and treatment of psoriasis: A review. JAMA. 2020;**323**(19):1945-1960

[3] Kamiya K et al. Risk factors for the development of psoriasis. International Journal of Molecular Sciences. 2019;**20**:1-14

[4] Ashcroft DM et al. Systematic review of comparative efficacy and tolerability of calcipotriol in treating chronic plaque psoriasis. BMJ. 2000;**320**:963-967

[5] Rendon A, Schakel K. Psoriasis pathogenesis and treatment. International Journal of Molecular Sciences. 2019;**20**:1475

[6] Kim WB, Jerome D, Yeung J. Diagnosis and management of psoriasis. Canadian Family Physician. 2017;**63**(4):278-285

[7] Langley R, Krueger G, Griffiths C. Psoriasis: Epidemiology, clinical features, and quality of life. Annals of the Rheumatic Diseases. 2005;**64**(suppl. 2):ii18-ii23

[8] Mihu C et al. Novel concepts in psoriasis: Histopathology and markers related to modern treatment approaches. Romanian Journal of Morphology and Embryology. 2021;**62**(4):897

[9] Ferrándiz C et al. Psoriasis of early and late onset: A clinical and epidemiologic study from Spain. Journal of the American Academy of Dermatology. 2002;**46**(6):867-873

[10] McBane S, Weigle N. Psoriasis. American Family Physician. 2013;**87**(9):626-633

[11] Griffiths CE, Barker JN. Pathogenesis and clinical features of psoriasis. The Lancet. 2007;**370**(9583):263-271

[12] Archid R et al. Relationship between histological and clinical course of psoriasis: A pilot investigation by reflectance confocal microscopy during Goeckerman treatment. Skin Pharmacology and Physiology. 2016;**29**(1):47-54

[13] Tsukazaki H, Kaito T. The role of the IL-23/IL-17 pathway in the pathogenesis of spondyloarthritis. International Journal of Molecular Sciences. 2020;**21**(17):6401

[14] Antonella D, Paola D, Frank O. The IL-23/Th17 axis in the immunopathogenesis of psoriasis. The Journal of Investigative Dermatology. 2009;**129**:1339-1331, 1350

[15] Stanway A. Guttate Psoriasis. 2021. Available from: https://dermnetnz.org/topics/guttate-psoriasis [Accessed: February 6, 2024]

[16] Daudén E et al. Long-term safety of nine systemic medications for psoriasis: A cohort study using the Spanish Registry of Adverse Events for Biological Therapy in Dermatological Diseases (BIOBADADERM) Registry. Journal of the American Academy of Dermatology. 2020;**83**(1):139-150

[17] Mehlis SL, Gordon KB. The immunology of psoriasis and biologic

immunotherapy. Journal of the American Academy of Dermatology. 2003;**49**(2):44-50

[18] Krueger JG. The immunologic basis for the treatment of psoriasis with new biologic agents. Journal of the American Academy of Dermatology. 2002;**46**(1):1-26

[19] Goolam Mahyoodeen N et al. High burden of the metabolic syndrome and its component disorders in South Africans with psoriasis. International Journal of Dermatology. 2019;**58**(5):557-562

[20] Parisi R et al. Global epidemiology of psoriasis: A systematic review of incidence and prevalence. Journal of Investigative Dermatology. 2013;**133**(2):377-385

[21] Pandey SS et al. Cyclosporine laden tailored microemulsion-gel depot for effective treatment of psoriasis: In vitro and in vivo studies. Colloids and Surfaces B: Biointerfaces. 2020;**186**:110681

[22] Choi CW et al. The advantage of cyclosporine A and methotrexate rotational therapy in long-term systemic treatment for chronic plaque psoriasis in a real world practice. Annals of Dermatology. 2017;**29**(1):55-60

[23] Springate D et al. Incidence, prevalence and mortality of patients with psoriasis: A UK population-based cohort study. British Journal of Dermatology. 2017;**176**(3):650-658

[24] Frez MLF et al. Recommendations for a patient-centered approach to the assessment and treatment of scalp psoriasis: A consensus statement from the Asia Scalp Psoriasis Study Group. Journal of Dermatological Treatment. 2014;**25**(1):38-45

[25] Raboobee N et al. Guidelines on the management of psoriasis in South Africa. South African Medical Journal. 2010;**100**(4):255-286

[26] Tucker LJ, Ye W, Coates LC. Novel concepts in psoriatic arthritis management: Can we treat to target? Current Rheumatology Reports. 2018;**20**:1-9

[27] Levine D, Gottlieb A. Evaluation and management of psoriasis: An internist's guide. Medical Clinics. 2009;**93**(6):1291-1303

[28] Michalek I, Loring B, John S. A systematic review of worldwide epidemiology of psoriasis. Journal of the European Academy of Dermatology and Venereology. 2017;**31**(2):205-212

[29] Lima X et al. Psoriasis prevalence among the 2009 AAD national melanoma/skin cancer screening program participants. Journal of the European Academy of Dermatology and Venereology. 2013;**27**(6):680-685

[30] Bowcock AM. The genetics of psoriasis and autoimmunity. Annual Review of Genomics and Human Genetics. 2005;**6**:93-122

[31] Hartshorne S. Dermatological disorders in Johannesburg, South Africa. Clinical and Experimental Dermatology. 2003;**28**(6):661-665

[32] Ammar-Khodja A et al. EPIMAG: International cross-sectional epidemiological psoriasis study in the Maghreb. Dermatology. 2015;**231**(2):134-144

[33] Griffiths PL et al. Socio-economic status and body composition outcomes in urban South African children. Archives of Disease in Childhood. 2008;**93**(10):862-867

[34] Alinaghi F et al. Prevalence of psoriatic arthritis in patients with psoriasis: A systematic review and meta-analysis of observational and clinical studies. Journal of the American Academy of Dermatology. 2019;**80**:251-256

[35] Henes JC et al. High prevalence of psoriatic arthritis in dermatological patients with psoriasis: A cross-sectional study. Rheumatology International. 2014;**34**:227-234

[36] Mease PJ. Measures of psoriatic arthritis: Tender and Swollen Joint Assessment, Psoriasis Area and Severity Index (PASI), Nail Psoriasis Severity Index (NAPSI), Modified Nail Psoriasis Severity Index (mNAPSI), Mander/Newcastle Enthesitis Index (MEI), Leeds Enthesitis Index (LEI), Spondyloarthritis Research Consortium of Canada (SPARCC), Maastricht Ankylosing Spondylitis Enthesis Score (MASES), Leeds Dactylitis Index (LDI), Patient Global for Psoriatic Arthritis, Dermatology Life Quality Index (DLQI), Psoriatic Arthritis Quality of Life (PsAQOL), Functional Assessment of Chronic Illness Therapy–Fatigue (FACIT-F), Psoriatic Arthritis Response Criteria (PsARC), Psoriatic Arthritis Joint Activity Index (PsAJAI), Disease Activity in Psoriatic Arthritis (DAPSA), and Composite Psoriatic Disease Activity Index (CPDAI). Arthritis Care & Research. 2011;**63**(S11):S64-S85

[37] Mease PJ et al. Prevalence of rheumatologist-diagnosed psoriatic arthritis in patients with psoriasis in European/North American dermatology clinics. Journal of the American Academy of Dermatology. 2013;**69**(5):729-735

[38] Villani AP et al. Prevalence of undiagnosed psoriatic arthritis among psoriasis patients: Systematic review and meta-analysis. Journal of the American Academy of Dermatology. 2015;**73**(2):242-248

[39] Cantatore FP et al. Angiogenesis dysregulation in psoriatic arthritis: Molecular mechanisms. BioMed Research International. 2017;**2017**

[40] Sakkas LI et al. Enthesitis in psoriatic arthritis. In: Seminars in Arthritis and Rheumatism. Elsevier; 2013:5312813

[41] Kataria RK, Brent LH. Spondyloarthropathies. American Family Physician. 2004;**69**(12):2853-2860

[42] Stoll ML et al. Patients with juvenile psoriatic arthritis comprise two distinct populations. Arthritis & Rheumatism: Official Journal of the American College of Rheumatology. 2006;**54**(11):3564-3572

[43] Pasch MC. Nail psoriasis: A review of treatment options. Drugs. 2016;**76**(6):675-705

[44] Maejima H et al. Evaluation of Nail Disease in Psoriatic Arthritis by Using a Modified Nail Psoriasis Severity Score Index. Wiley Online Library; 2010

[45] Langenbruch A et al. Nail involvement as a predictor of concomitant psoriatic arthritis in patients with psoriasis. British Journal of Dermatology. 2014;**171**(5):1123-1128

[46] Grewal S et al. The risk of IgA nephropathy and glomerular disease in patients with psoriasis: A population-based cohort study. British Journal of Dermatology. 2017;**176**(5):1366-1369

[47] Wan J et al. Risk of moderate to advanced kidney disease in patients with psoriasis: Population based cohort study. BMJ. 2013;**347**:f5961

[48] Yeung H et al. Psoriasis severity and the prevalence of major

medical comorbidity: A population-based study. JAMA Dermatology. 2013;**149**(10):1173-1179

[49] Ellinghaus D et al. Combined analysis of genome-wide association studies for Crohn disease and psoriasis identifies seven shared susceptibility loci. The American Journal of Human Genetics. 2012;**90**(4):636-647

[50] The Wellcome Trust Case Control Consortium. Genome-wide association study of 14,000 cases of seven common diseases and 3,000 shared controls. Nature. 2007;**447**(7145):661-678

[51] Azfar RS et al. The risk of stroke in patients with psoriasis. Journal of Investigative Dermatology. 2009;**129**:2411-2418

[52] Stern RS. Psoriasis is not a useful independent risk factor for cardiovascular disease. Journal of Investigative Dermatology. 2010;**130**:917-919

[53] Bao Y et al. Coronary heart disease and stroke risk in patients with psoriasis: Retrospective analysis. The American Journal of Medicine. 2010;**123**(4):350-357

[54] Armstrong A, Harskamp C, Armstrong E. The association between psoriasis and obesity: A systematic review and meta-analysis of observational studies. Nutrition & Diabetes. 2012;**2**(12):e54-e54

[55] Paroutoglou K et al. Deciphering the association between psoriasis and obesity: Current evidence and treatment considerations. Current Obesity Reports. 2020;**9**:165-178

[56] Chiricozzi A et al. Crosstalk between skin inflammation and adipose tissue-derived products: Pathogenic evidence linking psoriasis to increased adiposity. Expert Review of Clinical Immunology. 2016;**12**(12):1299-1308

[57] Johnston A et al. Obesity in psoriasis: Leptin and resistin as mediators of cutaneous inflammation. British Journal of Dermatology. 2008;**159**(2):342-350

[58] Galluzzo M et al. Bioelectrical impedance analysis to define an excess of body fat: Evaluation in patients with psoriasis. Journal of Dermatological Treatment. 2017;**28**(4):299-303

[59] Afach S et al. Systemic pharmacological treatments for chronic plaque psoriasis: A network meta-analysis. The Cochrane Database of Systematic Reviews. 2022;**5**:CD011535

[60] De Hoop D et al. Double-blinded, right/left comparison of calcipotriol and betamethasone valerate in treatment of psoriasis vulgaris. Lancet. 1991;**337**:193-196

[61] Mabuchi T, M. Tokuyama new treatment addressing the pathogenesis of psoriasis. International Journal of Molecular Sciences. 2020;**21**:7488

[62] Gardner SS. Psoriasis Treatment: When Should You Consider a Biologic. 2023. Available from: https://www.webmd.com/skin-problems-and-treatments/psoriasis/psoriasis-biologics

[63] Gudjonsson JE, Yost J. The role of TNF inhibitors in psoriasis therapy: New implications for associated comorbidities. F1000 Medicine Reports. 2009;**1**:30

[64] Grey H, Sellers AD. MNT Investigates: A Closer Look at IL-23 Inhibitors for Psoriasis. Medical news today; 2023. Available from: https://www.medicalnewstoday.com/articles/

il-23-inhibitors-for-psoriasis#side-effects [Accessed: February 06, 2024]

[65] Group W. The World Health Organization quality of life assessment (WHOQOL): Position paper from the World Health Organization. Social Science & Medicine. 1995;**41**(10):1403-1409

[66] Agrawal K, Singh S. Stress and psoriasis: An overview. The Pharma Innovation Journal. 2018;**7**(6):648-650

[67] Benhadou F, Mintoff D, Del Marmol V. Psoriasis: Keratinocytes or immune cells–which is the trigger? Dermatology. 2019;**235**(2):91-100

[68] Meneguin S et al. Quality of life of patients living with psoriasis: A qualitative study. BMC Dermatology. 2020;**20**(1):1-6

[69] Meher C, et al. Improving the quality of life in psoriasis patient through health promotion approach at Haji Adam Malik General Hospital, Medan. Asian Journal of Pharmaceutical and Clinical Research. 2018;**11**(10):107-110

[70] Naldi L et al. Cigarette smoking, body mass index, and stressful life events as risk factors for psoriasis: Results from an Italian case–control study. Journal of Investigative Dermatology. 2005;**125**(1):61-67

[71] Hayes J, Koo J. Psoriasis: Depression, anxiety, smoking, and drinking habits. Dermatologic Therapy. 2010;**23**(2):174-180

[72] Bilgic A et al. Psychiatric symptoms and health-related quality of life in children and adolescents with psoriasis. Pediatric Dermatology. 2010;**27**(6):614-617

[73] Gånemo A, Wahlgren CF, Svensson Å. Quality of life and clinical features in Swedish children with psoriasis. Pediatric Dermatology. 2011;**28**(4):375-379

[74] Hughes O, Hutchings PB, Phelps C. Stigma, social appearance anxiety and coping in men and women living with skin conditions: A mixed methods analysis. Skin Health and Disease. 2022;**2**(4):e73

[75] Chung J et al. Palmoplantar psoriasis is associated with greater impairment of health-related quality of life compared with moderate to severe plaque psoriasis. Journal of the American Academy of Dermatology. 2014;**71**(4):623-632

[76] Patel N et al. Psoriasis, depression, and inflammatory overlap: A review. American Journal of Clinical Dermatology. 2017;**18**(5):613-620

[77] Lakshmy S et al. A cross-sectional study of prevalence and implications of depression and anxiety in psoriasis. Indian Journal of Psychological Medicine. 2015;**37**(4):434-440

[78] Basavaraj KH, Navya MA, Rashmi R. Stress and quality of life in psoriasis: An update. International Journal of Dermatology. 2011;**50**(7):783-792

[79] Taborda M-LV, Weber MB, Freitas ES. Assessment of the prevalence of psychological distress in patients with psychocutaneous disorder dermatoses. Anais Brasileiros de Dermatologia. 2005;**80**:351-354

[80] Nguyen CM et al. The psychosocial impact of acne, vitiligo, and psoriasis: A review. Clinical, Cosmetic and Investigational Dermatology. 2016;**9**:383-392

[81] Janowski K et al. Social support and adaptation to the disease in

men and women with psoriasis. Archives of Dermatological Research. 2012;**304**:421-432

[82] Kaushik SB, Lebwohl MG. Review of safety and efficacy of approved systemic psoriasis therapies. International Journal of Dermatology. 2019;**58**(6):649-658

[83] Salman A et al. Impact of psoriasis in the quality of life of children, adolescents and their families: A cross-sectional study. Anais Brasileiros de Dermatologia. 2018;**93**:819-823

[84] Mrowietz U et al. Definition of treatment goals for moderate to severe psoriasis: A European consensus. Archives of Dermatological Research. 2011;**303**:1-10

[85] Honma M, Hayashi K. Psoriasis: Recent progress in molecular-targeted therapies. The Journal of Dermatology. 2021;**48**(6):761-777

[86] Kimball AB et al. The psychosocial burden of psoriasis. American Journal of Clinical Dermatology. 2005;**6**:383-392

[87] Fortune D et al. A cognitive-behavioural symptom management programme as an adjunct in psoriasis therapy. British Journal of Dermatology. 2002;**146**(3):458-465

[88] Safdari R, Firoz A, Masoorian H. Identifying training and informational components to develop a psoriasis self-management application. Medical Journal of the Islamic Republic of Iran. 2017;**31**:67

[89] Thorneloe RJ et al. Adherence to medication in patients with psoriasis: A systematic literature review. British Journal of Dermatology. 2013;**168**(1):20-31

[90] Bhosle MJ et al. Medication adherence and health care costs associated with biologics in Medicaid-enrolled patients with psoriasis. Journal of Dermatological Treatment. 2006;**17**(5):294-301

[91] Schmitt-Egenolf M. Physical Activity and Lifestyle Improvement in the Management of Psoriasis. Oxford, UK: Blackwell Publishing Ltd; 2016. pp. 452-453

[92] Katsurada E. A pilot study on the effect of massage on stress among female Japanese university students. Women Health Open Journal. 2019;**5**(1):1-5

[93] Coyle M et al. Acupuncture therapies for psoriasis vulgaris: A systematic review of randomized controlled trials. Complementary Medicine Research. 2015;**22**(2):102-109

[94] Stier-Jarmer M et al. Effects of single moor baths on physiological stress response and psychological state: A pilot study. International Journal of Biometeorology. 2017;**61**:1957-1964

[95] Spilioti E et al. Biological properties of mud extracts derived from various spa resorts. Environmental Geochemistry and Health. 2017;**39**:821-833

[96] Telles S et al. A critical evaluation of dead sea therapy in the management of psoriasis. Journal of Alternative Complementary and Integrative Medicine. 2017;**3**:15-17

[97] Wahedi HM et al. Aloesin from Aloe vera accelerates skin wound healing by modulating MAPK/Rho and Smad signaling pathways in vitro and in vivo. Phytomedicine. 2017;**28**:19-26

[98] Jankowiak B et al. Stigmatization and quality of life in patients with psoriasis. Dermatology and Therapy. 2020;**10**(2):285-296

[99] Goffman E. Stigma: Notes on the Management of Spoiled Identity. Simon and Schuster; 2009

[100] Topp J et al. Strategies to reduce stigma related to visible chronic skin diseases: A systematic review. Journal of the European Academy of Dermatology and Venereology. 2019;**33**(11):2029-2038

[101] Corker E et al. Experiences of discrimination among people using mental health services in England 2008-2011. The British Journal of Psychiatry. 2013;**202**(s55):s58-s63

[102] Weiss MG. Stigma and the social burden of neglected tropical diseases. PLoS Neglected Tropical Diseases. 2008;**2**(5):e237

[103] Picco L et al. Internalized stigma among psychiatric outpatients: Associations with quality of life, functioning, hope and self-esteem. Psychiatry Research. 2016;**246**:500-506

[104] Zięciak T et al. Feelings of stigmatization and depressive symptoms in psoriasis patients. Psychiatria Polska. 2017;**51**(6)

[105] Žarković Palijan T et al. The impact of psoriasis on the quality of life and psychological characteristics of persons suffering from psoriasis. Collegium Antropologicum. 2011;**35**(2):81-85

[106] Yang H-J, Yang K-C. Impact of psoriasis on quality of life in Taiwan. Dermatologica Sinica. 2015;**33**(3):146-150

[107] Strober B et al. Impact of psoriasis severity on patient-reported clinical symptoms, health-related quality of life and work productivity among US patients: Real-world data from the Corrona Psoriasis Registry. BMJ Open. 2019;**9**(4):e027535

[108] Agarwal K et al. Impact of psoriasis on quality of life. Indian Journal of Dermatology. 2022;**67**(4):387-391

[109] Armstrong AW et al. Quality of life and work productivity impairment among psoriasis patients: Findings from the National Psoriasis Foundation Survey Data 2003-2011. PLoS ONE. 2012;**7**(12):e52935

[110] Bewley A et al. Identifying individual psychosocial and adherence support needs in patients with psoriasis: A multinational two-stage qualitative and quantitative study. Journal of the European Academy of Dermatology and Venereology. 2014;**28**(6):763-770

[111] Kouris A et al. Quality of life and psychosocial aspects in Greek patients with psoriasis: A cross-sectional study. Anais Brasileiros de Dermatologia. 2015;**90**:841-845

[112] Obradors M et al. Health-related quality of life in patients with psoriasis: A systematic review of the European literature. Quality of Life Research. 2016;**25**(11):2739-2754

[113] Grozdev I et al. Physical and mental impact of psoriasis severity as measured by the compact short form-12 health survey (SF-12) quality of life tool. Journal of Investigative Dermatology. 2012;**132**(4):1111-1116

[114] Kilanowski JF. Breadth of the socio-ecological model. Journal of Agromedicine. 2017;**22**(4):295-297

[115] Tisdale RL et al. Patient-centered, sustainable hypertension care: The case for adopting a differentiated service delivery model for hypertension services in low-and middle-income countries. Global Heart. 2021;**16**(1)

Chapter 3

Psoriasis and Exposome: Unveiling the Inner and the External Contributors of Psoriasis Disease

Efterpi Zafiriou, Emmanouil Karampinis and Angeliki-Victoria Roussaki-Schulze

Abstract

The term "exposome" encompasses all the environmental elements, both infectious and non-infectious, that an individual encounters throughout life. It refers to the collective exposure to various factors in the environment that can have an impact on human health and finally result in a disease or affect the disease course. The exposome is a term implicated in all skin diseases including psoriasis. Ranging from lifestyle habits such as diet, smoking, obesity, sunlight exposure, pre-existing diseases, and infectious agents' exposure to patients' unique features such as skin microbes, oxidative stress parameters, skin chemical environment, and cutaneous immune reactions, skin seems to encounter a variety of different exposures. All these exposures in turn affect and contribute in distinct ways to the pathogenesis pathways implicated in the creation of the psoriatic skin lesions and shape the disease course and progression. Also, the interaction between environmental and genetic factors is a well-established disease contributor. This chapter discusses the link between each aspect of exposome and psoriasis pathways and mechanisms as well as treatment plans taking into consideration environmental factors. Understanding the exposome–psoriasis relationship would lead to implications and targeted interventions to mitigate possible risk factors and give future directions.

Keywords: psoriasis, exposome, environment, lifestyle, genetics, microbioma

1. Introduction

Psoriasis is a persistent skin disease caused by immune system dysfunction and manifests with various phenotypically distinct subtypes such as plaque, guttate, pustular, or erythrodermic psoriasis. The disease, in its plaque form, which is the most frequent subtype, is characterized by well-defined, reddish, scaly plaques resulting from increased keratinocyte proliferation and proinflammatory cytokines. All forms are linked with genetic contributors, whose products are mainly involved in skin immune reactions and skin barrier formation [1].

The exposome represents all environmental exposures, from infectious and non-infectious causes that can contribute to the disease onset, making the hypothesis that everyone's disease including psoriasis is the result of the individual history of exposures, considering the individual's genetic susceptibilities. Apart from environmental exposures (air pollution, sunlight exposure) and lifestyle aspects (diet, exercise), exposome concept encompasses psycho-social practices while its yields such as epigenomics, transcriptomics, proteomics, and metabolomics as disease mechanisms are in the spotlight [2].

The pathogenesis of psoriasis is multifactorial, combining environmental and genetic factors and necessitating a further exploration of the concept of exposome. When individuals with a genetic predisposition encounter triggers for psoriasis, the adaptive immune system sets off a cascade of immune responses. The immunological pathways, specifically the IL-17 signaling pathway and its products, play a crucial role in driving the inflammatory cycle of psoriasis. More precisely, the myeloid dendritic cells release IL-12 and IL-23, with the IL-23 pathway being the primary driver in psoriasis pathogenesis as this cytokine supports the survival, differentiation, and activation of Th17 cells, which produce IL-17 cytokines. These cytokines, in turn, induce keratinocyte proliferation and promote the production of various psoriasis-related cytokines, chemokines, inflammatory mediators, and antimicrobial peptides. Pinpointing the psoriasis triggers and understanding their impact on specific aspects of psoriasis pathophysiology can pave the way for preventive strategies and practical application of the exposome concept [1].

Additionally, the presence of a disrupted skin barrier with impaired permeability plays a crucial role in the development of psoriasis. In susceptible individuals, skin injury can trigger psoriatic lesions, a phenomenon called Koebner phenomenon [3]. This process is likely mediated by the injury prompting keratinocytes to produce type 1 interferons, TNF-α, IL-6, and IL-36. In psoriasis, skin barrier dysfunction is also linked to the disruption of epidermal tight, gap, and adherent junction proteins. The reduced expression of these proteins likely contributes to increased transepidermal water loss and decreased hydration observed in psoriatic lesions [3, 4]. Therefore, mechanical or external exposures can contribute to the disease because of the compromised skin barrier.

Psoriasis disease is evaluated by the extent of skin involvement (body surface area (BSA)) and the severity of erythema, induration, and scaling, resulting in disease assessment scores such as the Psoriasis Area Severity Index (PASI). Treatment options include topical therapies such as vitamin D analogs (calcipotriol) or corticosteroids as well as phototherapy, systemic agents (methotrexate, ciclosporin and acitretin) and biologics such as TNF (adalimumab, etanercept, infliximab and certolizumab), IL-12/23p40 (ustekinumab), IL-23p19 (rizankizumab, guselkumab and tildrakizumab), IL-17 (ixekizumab and secukinumab), and IL-17 receptor (brodalumab) inhibitors. The combination of the proper treatment choice and the limitations of the exposome's psoriasis modulatory factors can open new perspectives in the approach of psoriasis patients [1].

2. Inner contributors of psoriasis disease

The internal exposome pertains to individual-specific exposures within the body, encompassing genetic determinants, metabolic processes, and circulating blood biomarkers such as systematic oxidative stress parameters, hormones, and variability of skin as well as oral or gut microbiota [2].

2.1 Genetics and/or genomics of psoriasis

Basic principles: The evaluation of exposome factors affecting the onset of chronic diseases has focused on the analysis and the synergic effect with individual genetic variations induced by single-nucleotide polymorphism (SNP) and their associated proteome reactions. These genetic differences determine the patient's susceptibility to developing a disease when exposed to specific exposome factors [5]. Genomics is a term relating all genes and their interrelationships in order to identify their combined influence on the growth and development of psoriasis.

Exposome aspect—Disease pathophysiology link: Psoriasis risk has been associated with regions of the genome with critical genes involved in systemic and skin immunity as well as skin barrier formation [5]. Notably, those SNPs that represent genes variants of the above-mentioned genes have shown significant associations in psoriasis patients compared with controls. Worth mentioning are SNPs of genes whose products are involved in immune pathways, such as IL-17/IL-23 axis, type I interferon signaling, antigen-presenting process as well as nuclear factor-κB (NF-κB) pathways. In addition to susceptibility, those gene variants have been implicated in the time of onset, severity, comorbidities, and response to the treatment. However, those factors alone are not sufficient to predict the psoriasis disease course [6].

Clinical correlations: This section also has promising clinical correlations focused on personalized medicine as well as psoriasis-targeted therapies.

2.2 Oxidative stress parameters and psoriasis

Basic principles: Oxidative stress conditions are determined by the imbalance between the production and accumulation of oxygen reactive species (ROS) in cells and tissues and the body's ability by enzymatic and non-enzymatic mechanisms to detoxify these reactive substances. Under excessive oxidative stress, various cellular components, including membranes, lipids, proteins, lipoproteins, and deoxyribonucleic acid (DNA), are modified and lead to the formation of toxic and mutagenic products [7].

Exposome aspect—Disease pathophysiology link: UV radiation, air pollution, toxic substances, and their metabolites are responsible for the production of reactive oxygen and nitrogen species (ROS/RNS) [8]. ROS can also be produced due to polymorphisms of specific genes whose products regulate the redox balance and are often detected in psoriasis patients. ROS generated within the skin serves as chemo-attractants for neutrophils, which, in turn, can lead to further activation of neutrophils, creating a vicious circle [9]. Furthermore, oxidative stress promotes inflammation through several signaling pathways, mainly by NF-κB, that produce various cytokines and recruit additional inflammatory cells, leading to an augmented inflammatory response that preserves the chronic inflammatory nature of psoriasis [10].

Clinical correlations: Clinical correlations of oxidative stress are based on the assessment and comparison of *oxidative* stress parameters (toxic products, antioxidant enzyme activity, substrates of enzymatic reactions, etc.) in blood or tissue before and after an intervention or treatment initiation [11]. Skin and systematic oxidative stress have been implicated in many skin diseases including non-melanoma skin cancer [11]. In the study by Kökçam [12], the levels of glutathione (GSH), which is the most abundant antioxidant element in the cell and the activity of GSH-Px (GSH peroxidase) in both plasma and RBC samples were found lower in patients with psoriasis than in controls, whereas beta-carotene levels in plasma and MDA levels (lipid-oxidation parameter) in RBC samples were significantly higher in psoriasis patients, indicating higher systematic oxidative stress. Treatments for psoriasis, such as phototherapy and biologic systemic treatment, contribute to the induction of controlled oxidative stress, breaking the vicious circle between inflammation and oxidative stress [13]. An antioxidant diet including micronutrients such as polyphenols and carotenoids appears to have antioxidant characteristics with the following beneficial effect on skin [14], and topical application of antioxidants such as curcumin was proposed as an additional method to improve psoriasis disease's lesions [15].

2.3 Pre-existing conditions as a trigger factor of psoriasis

Basic principles: The exposome includes pre-existing conditions that might increase the likelihood of developing psoriasis. Psoriasis is linked with various coexisting medical conditions, including cardiovascular and mental health disorders as well as other diseases associated with systemic inflammation such as psoriatic arthritis, Crohn's disease, and ulcerative colitis [16].

Exposome aspect—Disease pathophysiology link: Increased levels of systemic inflammatory markers like C-reactive protein (CRP) may stem from interactions between proinflammatory cytokines IL-6, IL-1, and TNF-alpha. This elevation in inflammatory markers can potentially make patients more susceptible to experiencing negative cardiovascular events as well as developing psoriatic plaques. Regarding the link between skin and gut inflammation, Th17 cells in psoriatic skin produce IL-23, which is an essential cytokine for intestinal inflammation, leading to inflammatory bowel disease. In both instances, psoriasis can either be the initial diagnosed disease or occur subsequently. Depression and obesity will be discussed in the respective sections [16, 17].

Also, some medications used to treat specific diseases can lead to drug-induced psoriasis. For example, beta-blockers are widely prescribed for treating and preventing various medical conditions and block the beta-adrenergic subtype 2 receptors. As a result, adenyl cyclase is no longer activated, decreasing cAMP and intracellular calcium levels. This decrease disrupts the normal regulation of cell differentiation and promotes keratinocyte proliferation, which can have adverse effects on the skin [18].

Clinical correlations: It is crucial to conduct screenings for cardiovascular risk factors in psoriasis patients and, if heart disease is suspected, referred to the relevant specialists. Additionally, counseling patients on adopting healthy lifestyle habits such as proper diet, exercise, and smoking cessation is essential to minimize risk factors for comorbidities. Furthermore, the presence of concurrent diseases prompts specialists to adopt therapeutic approaches that do not negatively affect but benefit other systems [17].

2.4 Psoriasis and hormonal impact

Basic principles: Several studies examining the occurrence and severity of psoriasis in both genders indicated that psoriasis is more prevalent and severe in men compared to women, especially during periods of higher estrogen levels [19].

Exposome aspect—Disease pathophysiology link: Regarding sex hormones, estrogens inhibit the production of psoriasis-related cytokines like IL-1β and IL-23 by neutrophils and dendritic cells, respectively. However, in a psoriasis-control study, serum testosterone levels were significantly lower among psoriasis patients compared to control patients. It was also reported that testosterone promotes an immunological shift toward the Th2 phenotype [19]. Psoriasis severity in female patients can vary according to hormonal fluctuations, as psoriasis lesions tend to appear more frequently or worsen during puberty and improve during menopause. Pregnant women often experience complete resolution of psoriasis, but the condition may return after giving birth [20].

Thyroid hormones, specifically T3 (Triiodothyronine) and T4 (Thyroxine), trigger an elevation in epidermal growth factor (EGF) levels, resulting in epidermal hyperplasia or T3 itself promotes the proliferation of keratinocytes by T3 receptors on the skin. Stress, fast-modulation hormones, and circadian rhythm hormones will be discussed in the respective sections [21].

Clinical correlations: The immune-regulating effects of estrogen in psoriasis have been explored mainly *in vitro* studies. Additionally, findings from mouse psoriasis models indicated that targeted activation of estrogen receptor-signaling could be a promising new therapeutic approach for managing psoriasis, taking into consideration the adverse effects of estrogen therapy such as increased risk of thrombosis and endometrial cancer [19].

2.5 Metabolism profile (metabolics) in psoriasis patients

Basic principles: Metabolites directly reflect the biochemical processes occurring in a specific phenotype. They are the result-products of genomics and their associated proteomics and are closely linked to diseases and systemic conditions.

Exposome aspect—Disease pathophysiology link: In patients with psoriasis, insulin resistance and abnormal function of glucose transporter (GLUT) proteins have been observed, associated with susceptibility loci in metabolic diseases, including type 2 diabetes. Also, higher levels of α-ketoglutaric acid, lactic acid, aspartic acid, and glutamic acid are reported in psoriasis patients as these acids move in peripheral circulation and are consumed due to increased energy requirements related to cytokine production and rapid protein production due to cellular hyperproliferation. An excess of circulating free fatty acids can disrupt the β-pancreatic cell's normal function, leading to insulin resistance. Adipocytes also secrete multiple inflammation-associated cytokines, triggering various inflammatory responses. In psoriatic lesions, the levels of unsaturated fatty acids, some of which have anti-inflammatory effects and anti-proliferative properties, differ significantly. Dysregulation in urea circle and in phenylalanine-tyrosine pathway can produce more ornithine and phenylalanine levels in the psoriatic lesions. The rapid proliferation and differentiation of the epidermis in psoriasis patients lead to changes in nucleotide metabolism in the peripheral circulation. These alterations primarily manifest as reduced levels of certain metabolites due to the increased demand and hypercatabolism of purines and pyrimidines.

Clinical correlations: According to certain studies, elevated levels of amino acids involved in the both urea cycle and collagen synthesis (proline and hydroxyproline) in the bloodstream and in psoriatic lesions are believed to be linked to the severity of psoriasis and, therefore, new psoriasis markers can be introduced. Each patient has a different genetic and metabolic profile, and therefore, treatment strategies with metabolomics integration can lead to individualized therapies.

2.6 Microbiome (skin, oral, and gut) role in the development of psoriasis

Basic principles: Microbiome refers to the symbiotic microbial cells harbored by each person, encompassing primarily bacteria in the gut, skin, and oral cavity. The microbiome plays a vital role in regulating the immune system of the respective organ or tissue. Its imbalance, called dysbiosis, occurring in the skin and/or gut microbiome, is linked to altered immune responses, resulting in disease occurrence. The composition of the skin microbiome is determined by the individual's genetic factors as well as other exposome factors such as polymorphisms in filaggrin expression, hormonal factors, and variations in skin barrier function, indicating that one exposome factor can be influenced by the others, reinforcing the impact toward or against the onset of disease [22].

The skin and gut are heavily colonized by microbial cells, which in turn train the immune cells and determine the immunology capacity of the host. The gut–skin axis through the microbiome is a concept that has been referred to as skin disorders such as atopic dermatitis. The gut microbiome of infants with atopic dermatitis (AD) is characterized by lower levels of Bacteroidetes and Bifidobacterium and higher quantities of Clostridium and Escherichia, which, in turn, boost the inflammatory state in the intestine [23]. Those alterations in the gut microbiome disrupt the immune system balance by the production of inflammatory metabolites, which are released in the circulation and can affect skin. The Western diet and use of probiotics exacerbate and improve the skin manifestations of atopic dermatitis, respectively, indicating the existence of a skin-gut interaction, possibly by the microbiome [24].

Exposome aspect—Disease pathophysiology link: In case of psoriasis, the skin microbiome is mainly characterized by a relatively higher abundance of *Staphylococcus aureus* and *Streptococcus* species colonization and low quantities of immunoregulatory bacteria such as *Staphylococcus epidermidis* and *Propionibacterium acnes* [25]. This microbiome imbalance, mainly by *Staphylococcus aureus*, can trigger the production of IL-17 cytokine as defense mechanism of the skin. However, this IL-17 response fuels simultaneously pathogenic pathways of psoriasis. This microbiome imbalance exists both in psoriasis and not psoriasis lesions of the patient. Part of this microbial imbalance belongs to the decreased Actinobacteria-to-Firmicutes ratio, which is most prominent in skin lesions. Worth mentioning is that anti-psoriasis approaches such as UVB-light therapy and biology treatment change the microbiome diversity of the skin [26].

The skin-gut axis in psoriasis is not studied as deeply as in the case of atopic dermatitis. However, some structural variations have been reported, such as a decreased surface in the jejunum. This variation is responsible for differences in gut microbiome such as lower levels of Bacteroidetes and higher Firmicutes. Also, gut microbiome changes have been reported after biologic treatment such as secukinumab. Since the oral cavity is part of the gastrointestinal tract, a similar association is expected. An increased presence of oral Candida in patients with psoriasis has also been reported [23].

Clinical correlations-perspectives: A balanced skin microbiome helps to protect the skin from harmful pathogens and maintain its barrier function and therefore can be part of the psoriasis patient approach. The gut microbial composition and function are mainly influenced by dietary choices. Restoring the gut microbiome by diet, fecal transplants, and probiotics, can be used in patients with psoriasis and represent a promising preventive and therapeutic approach [23].

3. External contributors of psoriasis disease

The external contributors of exposome that promote psoriasis can be divided into general external factors (climate, biodiversity, urban environment, social, and economic elements) and specific external factors (infections, allergens, diet, tobacco, pollutants, and toxic substances) [27].

3.1 Environmental toxification and psoriasis disease

Basic principles: According to the 2019 Global Burden of Disease report, air pollution is the primary environmental risk factor for both adults and children. Carbon monoxide (CO), ozone (O_3), sulfur dioxide (SO_2), and nitrogen dioxide (NO_2) are among other monitored air pollutants due to their negative impact on health. When inhaled, these pollutants can enter the bloodstream, leading to oxidative damage and inflammation. Additionally, air pollutants can directly affect the skin upon contact [28].

Exposome aspect—Disease pathophysiology link: Bellinato et al. found that higher concentrations of different air pollutants were associated with psoriasis flares in patients living in an industrialized city [29]. Gaseous pollutants produce ROS and RNS species that overwhelm body's antioxidant defenses, causing higher cutaneous and systemic oxidative stress conditions leading to psoriasis. Among gas pollutants, NO_2 increased the risk of psoriasis occurrence. After inhalation, air pollutants can cause oxidative stress in the airway's epithelia but also reach peripheral tissues, such as skin, and due to oxidative stress—inflammation vicious circle, cause the production of proinflammatory cytokines that in turn are transferred into the bloodstream [30]. Also, direct skin contact with air pollutants can also add to the pathophysiology of psoriasis. Diesel exhaust particle exposure can trigger the activation of T cells present in the skin, leading to an abnormal release of proinflammatory cytokines such as TNF-α and interleukins (ILs) like IL-1 and IL-6 [29].

Clinical correlations—perspectives: It is crucial to understand that while pollutants can act as potential triggers and worsen psoriasis in some cases. Their impact, which seems to be unavoidable due to the industrialized way of everyday life, may vary among different individuals with psoriasis. Taking steps to minimize exposure to pollutants and adopting a healthy lifestyle can have positive effects on managing psoriasis and overall health.

3.2 Stress and psoriasis disease

Basic principles: Stress is widely recognized as a prominent trigger for psoriasis, and it has been linked with new onset as well as flare-ups of the disease. Psoriasis patients may experience anxiety because of the disease-related psychological burden of disfigurement, social stigmatization, or chronic itching. Furthermore, those stress feelings, along with dissatisfaction with treatment, may contribute to the development of depression in these individuals. Conversely, psoriasis can also be influenced or exacerbated by psychiatric conditions like depression and anxiety, creating a cyclical relationship [31].

Exposome aspect—Disease pathophysiology link: The pathogenesis link is based on the stress impact on immune function. Stress triggers the release of corticotropin-releasing hormone (CRH) in the hypothalamus, leading to elevated levels of adrenocorticotropic hormone (ACTH) in the bloodstream, which, in turn, induces the secretion of glucocorticoids (hypothalamic–pituitary–adrenal axis). CRH is also involved in the release of noradrenaline in the peripheral sympathetic nervous system and noradrenaline and adrenaline in the adrenal medulla, contributing to increased levels of neurohormones in the periphery. Immune system cells, such as T lymphocytes, B lymphocytes, and monocytes, express receptors for these hormones and therefore those cells' activation in peripheral organs such as the skin can lead to cutaneous inflammation and cause psoriasis flare [32, 33].

Elevated levels of cytokines have been observed in stress-related disorders, as indicated by a study involving medical students that connected psychological stress was associated with increased levels of cytokines [34]. Cytokines' levels were also assessed in psoriatic patients exposed to psychological stress. The salivary levels of IL-1β after stress stimuli were compared between psoriasis patients and control. Interestingly, after the stressful event, the control group showed an increase in IL-1β levels, while the psoriasis group did not, indicating an impaired immune system response to adrenergic stimuli [35]. However, this observation is not in line with the cytokine-mediated psoriasis flare-up that may be induced by stress.

In addition to acute experience of stress, chronic stress as well as depression has been linked to persistently high levels of proinflammatory cytokines, notably IL-6, TNF-α, and IL-1β. IL-6 and TNF-α can alter the metabolism of neurotransmitters like norepinephrine, serotonin, and dopamine, leading to depressive symptoms. Additionally, IL-6 promotes the production of Th17 cells and along with action of TNF-α, plays a central role in the development of psoriasis lesions [31, 32]. Additionally, the reduced levels of serotonin (5-HT) lead to increased production of certain inflammatory mediators like TNF-α and IL-1β [36].

Clinical correlations—perspectives: In clinical practice, those findings can be exploited by the development of drugs influencing the serotonergic and adrenergic systems to maintain the circulating levels of respective hormones to avoid a psoriasis flare-up. Research has already proved that anti-depressants have a protective effect on the risk of psoriasis in patients with Major Depressive Disorder. Individuals using antidepressants had a significantly lower risk of psoriasis compared to those who did not. Finally, further analysis revealed that the use of SSRIs (Selective Serotonin Reuptake Inhibitors) and lower dosages of antidepressants were associated with a statistically significant decrease in the risk of psoriasis [37].

3.3 Sleep habits and psoriasis-circadian rhythm

Basic principles: The circadian system comprises the master clock in the suprachiasmatic nucleus of the brain, serving as the central pacemaker and which regulates the daily rhythm of the other organs. An example of circadian rhythm is that of cardiovascular system, as there is a reduction in vascular tone and blood coagulability at night [38].

As for the skin, the pineal gland produces melatonin, which is a crucial regulator of the circadian balance. Melatonin levels follow the circadian rhythm, peaking at night and decreasing during the day. When exposed to light, melatonin levels promptly decline due to feedback inhibition, reducing its production. Melatonin is associated with hair growth, protection against ultraviolet (UV) damage in skin cells, wound healing, and antitumor effects [39].

Exposome aspect—Disease pathophysiology link: Psoriasis exhibits classical rhythmicity, with disease flares and associated symptoms such as itch and pruritus being more severe in the evening and worsening at night. The circadian clock plays a vital role in regulating various aspects of the immune system, and any disruption to this rhythm, whether through genetic alterations of central and peripheral regulators-components or changes in light-dark phases, significantly impacts immune response. Sleep deprivation resulted in increased levels of proinflammatory cytokines, including IL-1β, IL-6, and IL-12, leading to an intensified inflammatory immune response. This suggests that circadian disruption might contribute to the development and progression of psoriasis [38, 40].

Also, sleep loss is associated with function of the hypothalamic–pituitary–adrenal (HPA) axis, leading to psoriasis flare-ups as indicated in the stress-exposome, with increased secretion of cortisol and proinflammatory cytokines [38].

Clinical correlations—perspectives: The understanding of this exposome—parameter would lead to the identification of further intervention and enable targeted and personalized timing of psoriasis therapy to maximize treatment efficacy [40].

3.4 Diet and psoriasis

Basic principles: Diet plays a significant role in forming the composition of the gut microbiota, and therefore, the gut–skin axis discussed previously can affect the course of many skin disorders [41].

Exposome aspect—Disease pathophysiology link: Epidemiological studies have indicated that individuals with psoriasis had imbalanced dietary patterns, characterized by increased consumption of total fat and simple carbohydrates, which have been associated with activation of tumor necrosis factor-α/interleukin-23/interleukin-17 pathways, reactive oxygen species, and leukotrienes production and gut dysbiosis. Additionally, the diet that psoriasis patients usually adopt is characterized by reduced intake of proteins, complex carbohydrates, monounsaturated fatty acids, n-3 polyunsaturated fatty acids, vegetables, and fibers. This category of nutrients leads to the suppression of inflammatory pathways or induction of regulatory T cells, reducing the potential of inflammatory stimuli that can trigger psoriasis plaque formations [41, 42]. Worth mentioning is the lower intake of Mediterranean elements of nutrition (extra virgin olive oil, fruits, fish, and nuts) reported in psoriasis patients compared to healthy individuals. On the contrary, the Western diet has been accused of being a factor contributing to psoriasis. Indeed, after a short-term (4 weeks) exposure to a Western diet, there was an increase in the accumulation of IL-17 cells with enhanced expression of IL-23 receptors in imiquimod-induced psoriasiform dermatitis in murine models [41, 43].

Finally, the connection between obesity and psoriasis is well-established. As obesity progresses, adipocytes undergo senescence and dysfunction, altering their proteomic programming toward a proinflammatory phenotype. This shift may significantly influence the immune system's function and serve as a critical factor in the development of various organ pathologies including the skin, as far as the skin is concerned, and cause chronic inflammation. Gut dysbiosis and microbiome dysregulation as well as lipid signaling are involved in the inflammatory process [42, 44]. Notably, individuals with a body mass index (BMI) of 35 or higher demonstrated an increase in the risk of developing psoriasis in women population [45].

Clinical correlations—perspectives: The manipulation of gut microbiota, for example, by targeted introduction of specific live organisms with probiotics, offers promising new possibilities in managing various immune-related conditions characterized by uncontrolled inflammation. Antioxidant and anti-inflammatory nutrients such as phenolic compounds have also been extensively studied and have shown significant potential in treating skin diseases like psoriasis. Additionally, emerging therapies such as bariatric surgery, in case of obesity, have a substantial impact on the therapeutic approach to an obesity-psoriasis patient. These advancements hold great promise for the future management of combined immune-related skin disorders such as psoriasis and obesity [46].

3.5 Exercise and psoriasis

Basic principles: Regular physical exercise, such as activities like walking, dancing, yoga, skiing, and gardening, plays a vital role in regulating the levels of ROS and RNS in cells, species that control the balance between the normal cellular adaptation to keep their homeostasis and, in case of excessive production and accumulation leading to high oxidative stress conditions and disease. Also, regular exercise enhances the functioning of the immune system by reducing adiposity and its associated inflammatory inducement. Moreover, exercise has been found to have beneficial effects on mental health, reducing psychological stress, anxiety, and depression [47, 48].

Exposome aspect—Disease pathophysiology link: Regular exercise reduces fat mass, which can subsequently reduce its contribution to systemic inflammation and, due to the brain–skin axis, can reduce stress and its impact on skin. The proposal of the authors regarding the amount of exercise to reduce the risk of psoriasis flare differs [48]. Goto et al. proposed that less than 1 hour of exercise per week was associated with incident psoriasis [49], while Frankel et al. concluded that the most active quintile had a lower risk of developing psoriasis compared to the least active quintile. Vigorous activity is also associated with a reduced risk of psoriasis [50].

Clinical correlations—perspectives: Engaging in exercise could serve as a beneficial preventive measure for psoriasis and may have the potential to improve the condition in overweight patients [48].

3.6 Sun exposure and psoriasis

Basic principles: Sunlight is composed of a spectrum of radiations that span from infrared to visible and UV light. The most well-known advantage of sun exposure is the synthesis of vitamin D, which is important for several physiological functions, especially maintenance of an adequate bone mineral density [51].

Exposome aspect—Disease pathophysiology link: UV radiation can modify the cytokine profile linked to psoriasis by steering the immune response away from the proinflammatory Th1/Th17 axis. The seasonal variation's impact on the course of psoriasis is well known, with many cases experiencing relief during summer and exacerbation during winter. Some individuals reported worsening of their psoriasis due to photosensitivity. Also, UV radiation, especially UVB, leads to vitamin D production in the skin. Vitamin D can enhance the synthesis of anti-inflammatory cytokines by suppressing or inhibiting the production of proinflammatory cytokines like IL-6 and TNF-α, which are involved in the pathogenesis of psoriatic skin. As a result, vitamin D may have a considerable impact on the chronic autoimmune or inflammatory aspects of the disease [51]. Finally, there is a study that reports that vitamin D sufficiency acts as a protective factor against psoriasis flare-ups when a triggering factor occurs such as COVID-19 vaccination [52].

Clinical correlations—perspectives: Psoriasis patients can benefit from sun exposure as it can have positive effects on their skin condition. However, this also raises concerns about the increased risk of skin cancer in these individuals. Vitamin D supplements have been suggested as a potential method to improve psoriasis, but their effectiveness has not been conclusively demonstrated.

3.7 Alcohol and tobacco abuse

Basic principles: Nicotine is the primary alkaloid found in tobacco, and it is responsible for the addictive properties of tobacco products. Nicotine is rapidly absorbed not only through the alveolar spaces in the lungs but also through the skin and intestinal mucosa. The liver primarily metabolizes nicotine into several active metabolites. Nicotine interacts with different subtypes of nicotinic acetylcholine receptors, which are not only present in the nervous system and adrenal medulla but also in various other tissues, including skin keratinocytes and inflammatory cells like monocytes and dendritic cells, promoting inflammatory process. Apart from nicotine, tobacco consists of over 7000 chemicals, and smoking is known to be a risk factor for various human diseases [53].

Another abuse form that needs to be highlighted is alcohol consumption. Ethanol can affect cutaneous skin barrier as well as cutaneous immune reactions. Also, alcohol consumption is related to many other disorders such as obesity, depression, and liver disorders that can further exacerbate any skin disorder [54].

Exposome aspect—Disease pathophysiology link: Smoking induces oxidative stress and the generation of harmful free radicals, which disrupt signal pathways relevant to psoriasis, such as the NF-κB and JAK–STAT pathways. Moreover, nicotine stimulates the increased secretion of various cytokines such as (IL)-12, TNF, and IL-2, which play crucial roles in psoriasis pathogenesis. Furthermore, it has been observed that smoking can also influence the expression of vascular endothelial growth factor, an essential factor in angiogenesis. Although the risk of psoriasis in subjects with a smoking duration of <10 years was almost the same as that of nonsmokers, a smoking duration ≥30 years led to twice the risk of psoriasis compared to nonsmokers individuals [55, 56].

Ethanol can be detected within human skin, being secreted by eccrine glands, mainly sweat glands, or through passive diffusion, and by its metabolites can enhance the proliferation and mRNA expression of proliferation-associated genes of keratinocytes, disrupting the skin's barrier function and increasing its permeability. Moreover, alcohol also affects lipid metabolism, affecting the lipid composition of the skin barrier. Also, the metabolism of ethanol is associated with the production of ROS. As a result, both ethanol and the produced ROS formed during ethanol metabolism generate an inflammatory environment and trigger psoriasis by regulating different signal transduction pathways and inducing the production of various proinflammatory cytokines in lymphocytes, macrophages, and keratinocytes [54].

Clinical correlations—perspectives: Quitting smoking could be a significant goal in preventing and managing psoriasis by ceasing smoking. The level of smoke-induced inflammation might decrease, either through a reduction in circulating inflammatory cytokines or the restoration of T-cell impairments. Patients with psoriasis should receive counseling regarding the restricted use of alcohol, as it is associated with a higher risk of worsening the disease and its related comorbidities. Additionally, considering the potential impact of alcohol on concurrent pharmaceutical medications is important (avoidance of the combination of methotrexate and alcohol consumption due to risk for liver damage) [54, 57].

3.8 Mechanical trigger of psoriasis lesions

Basic principles: Several research studies emphasize the influence of mechanical forces and mechano-transduction in the initiation of the disease, leading to the activation of inflammation signaling pathways in keratinocytes [58].

Exposome aspect—Disease pathophysiology link: A typical example, widely known as Koebner phenomenon, involves the development of psoriatic plaques in apparently healthy skin following trauma and/or mechanical stress (scratches, abrasion, pressure from tight shoes, shaving, etc.). In case of psoriasis, the normal mechano-induced signaling pathways and molecules that translate mechanical forces to biochemical signals seem to be impaired (dysfunctional ion channels, protein pathways, and resulting abnormal destruction of tight junctions) [58].

Tattooing involves permanently marking the body with exogenous pigments or dyes introduced into the dermis for artistic purposes. The Koebner phenomenon, where psoriatic lesions develop at the site of skin trauma, has been documented in several case reports and one case series of patients with psoriasis who had tattoos [59].

Clinical correlations—perspectives: The exploration of mechano-transduction and mechano-sensing mechanisms is not adequately studied and, in case of psoriasis, can offer potential opportunities for identifying novel therapeutic targets [58].

3.9 Psoriasis and infectomics

Basic principles: Infection serves as an external trigger for psoriasis, as indicated by the well-established connection between the guttate psoriasis and acute streptococcal infection. Various infectious agents as the bacterium *Helicobacter pylori*, the fungi species Malassezia and Candida, as well as viral infections like human immunodeficiency virus (HIV), human papillomavirus (HPV), and hepatitis C virus (HCV) infection, along with the mite species Sarcoptidae are considered to be possible infectious triggers of psoriasis. Those infections seem to affect the immune cells, producing inflammatory cytokines that can initiate or worsen psoriasis [60, 61].

Exposome aspect—Disease pathophysiology link: Superantigens represent a classical mechanism by which bacteria can contribute to the formation of a psoriatic plaque. The connection between the outer surface of MHC class II proteins on antigen-presenting cells and T-cell receptors on the surface of T helper cells leads to their proliferation and cytokine production, such as IFN-γ. Additionally, superantigens enhance T-cell expression, promoting Th17-dominated responses and contributing to the pathogenesis of psoriasis [62].

In case of streptococcal infections and other Gram-positive organisms, the streptococcal cell wall is predominantly composed of peptidoglycan (PG), which is regarded as a potentially proinflammatory element and, therefore, another psoriasis mechanism can be observed besides superantigen action [63]. Additionally, serum anti-*Helicobacter pylori* immunoglobulin G (IgG) has been reported to be high in psoriasis patients, and their levels are connected with severity or duration of the disease [64, 65]. In case of viral hepatitis and HIV infection, common pathophysiology links have been reported such as the overproduction of TNF-α in HCV and changes in the constitution of lymphocyte subpopulations [66]. Psoriasis exacerbations and new onsets as well as new subtype psoriasis occurrences (such as pustular form in a patient with plaque psoriasis [67]) have been documented in case of COVID-19 infections and post-COVID-19 vaccinations [68]. The etiology proposed was the hyperinflammation state in both cases. Fungal infections, such as Malassezia and Candida, can predispose to psoriasis by Th1/Th2 cytokine imbalance and superantigen reaction, respectively [61].

Clinical correlations: Treatment options like antibiotics or tonsillectomy have been suggested for guttate psoriasis and flare-ups of chronic plaque psoriasis. The association between antibiotics and psoriasis has been a topic of discussion for many years, with reports of improvement, onset, or worsening of psoriasis observed after antibiotic treatment [61].

4. Discussion

The exposome is a complex area of scientific research that profoundly influences health. This concept provides a comprehensive understanding of the various exposures individuals encounter during their lifetime including internal and external environmental factors that can influence the onset and progression of specific diseases. Some aspects of the exposome, particularly external contributors, can be modified, such as quitting smoking, leading to potential positive effects on the disease [2]. Also, some external contributors can ameliorate the disease, such as sunlight-induced cutaneous immunosuppression [51].

Clinical perspectives on the exposome and the integration of internal factors like genomics with external contributors like diet are crucial in personalized medicine, promising a better approach to treating patients with psoriasis. Moreover, external exposure factors can trigger disease onset directly, as seen in the case of unhealthy diets which cause systemic inflammation and trigger psoriasis mechanisms. Additionally, these external factors can modify internal exposome factors, as a high-fat diet can lead to gut dysbiosis, which can worsen psoriasis through the gut–skin axis. The interaction between internal and external exposome factors plays a significant role in the development of psoriatic disease, with combinations like exercise-induced oxidative stress and stress-induced hormonal impacts (**Figure 1**). The result of those combinations as well as the direct effect of external and internal contributors can lead to systemic and cutaneous inflammation, leading to psoriasis (**Figure 1**). Understanding this interplay is of utmost importance in comprehending the complexities of psoriasis.

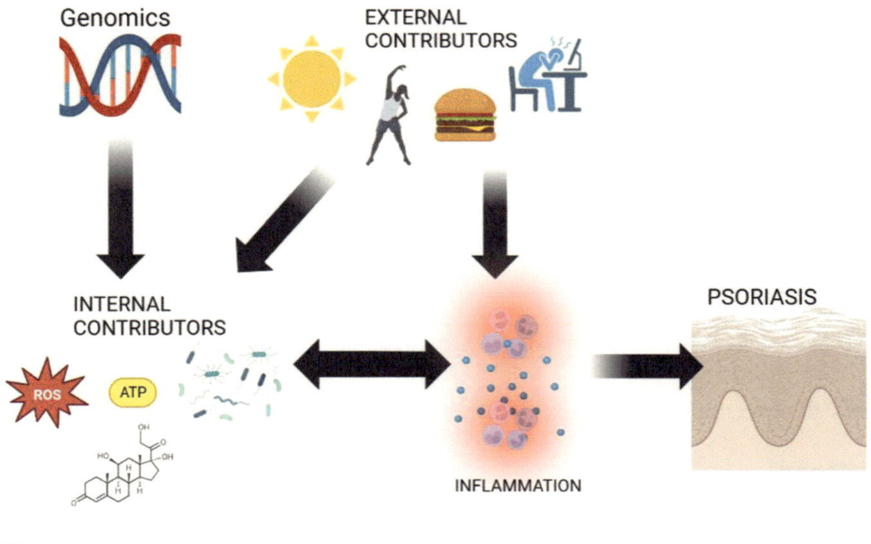

Figure 1.
The interaction between genomics, other internal contributors of exposome (oxidative stress parameters, metabolics, microbioma, hormonal impact), external contributors (sunlight, exercise, diet and stress), and main pathogenesis of psoriasis disease (skin inflammation) by single or bidirectional pathways (created by biorender.com).

However, some questions arise on whether an exposome variant is adequate for the expression of a disease phenotype or whether genomics is the indispensable inner contributor. A study showed that polymorphisms of the glutamate cysteine ligase catalytic subunit that regulates glutathione biosynthesis (GCLC) combined with tobacco smoking and alcohol abuse are significantly associated with the risk of psoriasis and related to its clinical features [69].

Also, the impact of exposomes on psoriasis disease seems to depend on the psoriasis stage. During the initiation stage, new inflammatory lesions continually emerge, while during the stationary stage, the lesions stabilize. Also, early and chronic psoriasis diseases differ in terms of immunology. In the initiation stage, the IL-23/IL-17 axis and activated DCs are the main contributors to the disease, while in chronic disease, mature dermal DCs and T cells contribute to the cytokine milieu [1]. Therefore, the result of exposome factors depends on the psoriasis stage. Also, the treatment status of psoriasis patients can defend against the psoriasis-provoking actions of some exposome factors. For example, patients under biologic treatment showed less frequent episodes of psoriasis flare-up following COVID-19 vaccination [67].

5. Conclusion

Exposome represents a multifaceted area of research that significantly impacts our understanding of psoriasis. This concept provides a comprehensive view of how various internal and external environmental factors interact to influence the onset and progression of psoriatic disease. More research in exposome in psoriasis disease is needed as its further exploration may open exciting possibilities for personalized medicine and targeted therapies.

Conflict of interest

The authors declare no conflict of interest.

Author details

Efterpi Zafiriou*, Emmanouil Karampinis and Angeliki-Victoria Roussaki-Schulze
Faculty of Medicine, School of Health Sciences, Department of Dermatology, University General Hospital of Larissa, University of Thessaly, Larissa, Greece

*Address all correspondence to: zafevi@o365.uth.gr

References

[1] Rendon A, Schäkel K. Psoriasis pathogenesis and treatment. International Journal of Molecular Sciences. 2019;**20**:1475

[2] Wild CP. The exposome: From concept to utility. International Journal of Epidemiology. 2012;**41**:24-32

[3] Orsmond A, Bereza-Malcolm L, Lynch T, March L, Xue M. Skin barrier dysregulation in psoriasis. International Journal of Molecular Sciences. 2021;**22**:10841

[4] Montero-Vilchez T, Segura-Fernández-Nogueras M-V, Pérez-Rodríguez I, Soler-Gongora M, Martinez-Lopez A, Fernández-González A, et al. Skin barrier function in psoriasis and atopic dermatitis: Transepidermal water loss and temperature as useful tools to assess disease severity. Journal of Clinical Medicine. 2021;**10**:359

[5] Capon F. The genetic basis of psoriasis. International Journal of Molecular Sciences. 2017;**18**:2526

[6] Villarreal-Martinez A, Gallerdo-Blanco H, Cerda-Flores R, Torres-Munoz I, Gomez-Flores M, Salas-Alanis J, et al. Candidate gene polymorphisms and risk of psoriasis: A pilot study. Experimental and Therapeutic Medicine. 2016;**11**:1217-1222

[7] Pizzino G, Irrera N, Cucinotta M, Pallio G, Mannino F, Arcoraci V, et al. Oxidative stress: Harms and benefits for human health. Oxidative Medicine and Cellular Longevity. 2017;**2017**:1-13

[8] Pleńkowska J, Gabig-Cimińska M, Mozolewski P. Oxidative stress as an important contributor to the pathogenesis of psoriasis. International Journal of Molecular Sciences. 2020;**21**:6206

[9] Vorobjeva N, Prikhodko A, Galkin I, Pletjushkina O, Zinovkin R, Sud'ina G, et al. Mitochondrial reactive oxygen species are involved in chemoattractant-induced oxidative burst and degranulation of human neutrophils in vitro. European Journal of Cell Biology. 2017;**96**:254-265

[10] Goldminz AM, Au SC, Kim N, Gottlieb AB, Lizzul PF. NF-κB: An essential transcription factor in psoriasis. Journal of Dermatological Science. 2013;**69**:89-94

[11] Karampinis E, Aloizou A-M, Zafiriou E, Bargiota A, Skaperda Z, Kouretas D, et al. Non-melanoma skin cancer and vitamin D: The "lost sunlight" paradox and the oxidative stress explanation. Antioxidants. 2023;**12**:1107

[12] Kökçam İ, Nazıroğlu M. Antioxidants and lipid peroxidation status in the blood of patients with psoriasis. Clinica Chimica Acta. 1999;**289**:23-31

[13] Medovic MV, Jakovljevic VLJ, Zivkovic VI, Jeremic NS, Jeremic JN, Bolevich SB, et al. Psoriasis between autoimmunity and oxidative stress: Changes induced by different therapeutic approaches. Oxidative Medicine and Cellular Longevity. 2022;**2022**:1-17

[14] Katsimbri P, Korakas E, Kountouri A, Ikonomidis I, Tsougos E, Vlachos D, et al. The effect of antioxidant and anti-inflammatory capacity of diet on psoriasis and psoriatic arthritis phenotype: Nutrition as therapeutic tool? Antioxidants. 2021;**10**:157

[15] Guarneri F, Bertino L, Pioggia G, Casciaro M, Gangemi S. Therapies with antioxidant potential in psoriasis, vitiligo, and lichen planus. Antioxidants. 2021;**10**:1087

[16] de de Oliveira MFSP, de Rocha BO, Duarte GV. Psoriasis: Classical and emerging comorbidities. Anais Brasileiros de Dermatologia. 2015;**90**:9-20

[17] Daugaard C, Iversen L, Hjuler KF. Comorbidity in adult psoriasis: Considerations for the clinician. Psoriasis: Targets and Therapy. 2022;**12**:139-150

[18] Awad VM, Sakhamuru S, Kambampati S, Wasim S, Malik BH. Mechanisms of beta-blocker induced psoriasis, and psoriasis de novo at the cellular level. Cureus. 2020;**12**

[19] Adachi A, Honda T. Regulatory roles of estrogens in psoriasis. Journal of Clinical Medicine. 2022;**11**:4890

[20] Ceovic R, Mance M, Bukvic Mokos Z, Svetec M, Kostovic K, Stulhofer BD. Psoriasis: Female skin changes in various hormonal stages throughout life—Puberty, pregnancy, and menopause. BioMed Research International. 2013;**2013**:1-6

[21] Sweta K, Mm F, Lenin M. The putative role of thyroid hormones and vitamin D on severity and quality of life in psoriasis. International Journal of Applied & Basic Medical Research. 2020;**10**:173

[22] Carmona-Cruz S, Orozco-Covarrubias L, Sáez-de-Ocariz M. The human skin microbiome in selected cutaneous diseases. Frontiers in Cellular and Infection Microbiology. 2022;**12**

[23] De Pessemier B, Grine L, Debaere M, Maes A, Paetzold B, Callewaert C. Gut–skin axis: Current knowledge of the interrelationship between microbial dysbiosis and skin conditions. Microorganisms. 2021;**9**:353

[24] Hrestak D, Matijašić M, Čipčić Paljetak H, Ledić Drvar D, Ljubojević Hadžavdić S, Perić M. Skin microbiota in atopic dermatitis. International Journal of Molecular Sciences. 2022;**23**:3503

[25] Langan EA, Künstner A, Miodovnik M, Zillikens D, Thaçi D, Baines JF, et al. Combined culture and metagenomic analyses reveal significant shifts in the composition of the cutaneous microbiome in psoriasis. British Journal of Dermatology. 2019;**181**:1254-1264

[26] Chang H-W, Yan D, Singh R, Liu J, Lu X, Ucmak D, et al. Alteration of the cutaneous microbiome in psoriasis and potential role in Th17 polarization. Microbiome. 2018;**6**:154

[27] Celebi, Sozener Z, Özbey Yücel Ü, Altiner S, Ozdel Oztürk B, Cerci P, Türk M, et al. The external exposome and allergies: From the perspective of the epithelial barrier hypothesis. Frontiers in Allergy. 2022;**3**

[28] Koohgoli R, Hudson L, Naidoo K, Wilkinson S, Chavan B, Birch-Machin MA. Bad air gets under your skin. Experimental Dermatology. 2017;**26**:384-387

[29] Bellinato F, Adami G, Vaienti S, Benini C, Gatti D, Idolazzi L, et al. Association between short-term exposure to environmental air pollution and psoriasis flare. JAMA Dermatology. 2022;**158**:375

[30] Wang T, Xia Y, Zhang X, Qiao N, Ke S, Fang Q, et al. Short-term effects of air pollutants on outpatients with psoriasis in a Chinese city with a subtropical monsoon climate. Frontiers in Public Health. 2022;**10**

[31] Alesci A, Lauriano ER, Fumia A, Irrera N, Mastrantonio E, Vaccaro M, et al. Relationship between immune cells, depression, stress, and psoriasis: Could the use of natural products be helpful? Molecules. 2022;**27**:1953

[32] Rousset L, Halioua B. Stress and psoriasis. International Journal of Dermatology. 2018;**57**:1165-1172

[33] Tampa M, Sarbu M-I, Mitran M-I, Mitran C-I, Matei C, Georgescu S-R. The pathophysiological mechanisms and the quest for biomarkers in psoriasis, a stress-related skin disease. Disease Markers. 2018;**2018**:1-14

[34] Maes M, Song C, Lin A, De Jongh R, Van Gastel A, Kenis G, et al. The effects of psychological stress on humans: Increased production of pro-inflammatory cytokines and TH1-like response in stress-induced anxiety. Cytokine. 1998;**10**:313-318

[35] Mastrolonardo M, Alicino D, Zefferino R, Pasquini P, Picardi A. Effect of psychological stress on salivary interleukin-1β in psoriasis. Archives of Medical Research. 2007;**38**:206-211

[36] Wardhana M, Windari M, Puspasari N, Suryawati N. Role of serotonin and dopamine in psoriasis: A case-control study. Open Access Macedonian Journal of Medical Sciences. 2019;**7**:1138-1142

[37] Tzeng Y-M, Li I-H, Kao H-H, Shih J-H, Yeh C-B, Chen Y-H, et al. Protective effects of anti-depressants against the subsequent development of psoriasis in patients with major depressive disorder: A cohort study. Journal of Affective Disorders. 2021;**281**:590-596

[38] Nowowiejska J, Baran A, Flisiak I. Mutual relationship between sleep disorders, quality of life and psychosocial aspects in patients with psoriasis. Frontiers in Psychiatry. 2021;**12**

[39] Lyons AB, Moy L, Moy R, Tung R. Circadian rhythm and the skin: A review of the literature. The Journal of Clinical and Aesthetic Dermatology. 2019;**12**:42-45

[40] Luengas-Martinez A, Paus R, Iqbal M, Bailey L, Ray DW, Young HS. Circadian rhythms in psoriasis and the potential of chronotherapy in psoriasis management. Experimental Dermatology. 2022;**31**:1800-1809

[41] Kanda N, Hoashi T, Saeki H. Nutrition and psoriasis. International Journal of Molecular Sciences. 2020;**21**:5405

[42] Barros G, Duran P, Vera I, Bermúdez V. Exploring the links between obesity and psoriasis: A comprehensive review. International Journal of Molecular Sciences. 2022;**23**:7499

[43] Shi Z, Wu X, Yu S, Huynh M, Jena PK, Nguyen M, et al. Short-term exposure to a Western diet induces Psoriasiform dermatitis by promoting accumulation of IL-17A–producing γδ T cells. Journal of Investigative Dermatology. 2020;**140**:1815-1823

[44] Jensen P, Skov L. Psoriasis and obesity. Dermatology. 2016;**232**:633-639

[45] Setty AR. Obesity, waist circumference, weight change, and the risk of psoriasis in women. Archives of Internal Medicine. 2007;**167**:1670

[46] Villarreal-Calderón JR, Cuéllar RX, Ramos-González MR, Rubio-Infante N, Castillo EC, Elizondo-Montemayor L, et al. Interplay between the adaptive immune system and insulin resistance in weight loss induced by bariatric surgery. Oxidative Medicine and Cellular Longevity. 2019;**2019**:1-14

[47] Duchnik E, Kruk J, Tuchowska A, Marchlewicz M. The impact of diet

and physical activity on psoriasis: A narrative review of the current evidence. Nutrients. 2023;**15**:840

[48] Yeroushalmi S, Hakimi M, Chung M, Bartholomew E, Bhutani T, Liao W. Psoriasis and exercise: A review. Psoriasis (Auckland, N.Z.). 2022;**12**:189-197

[49] Goto H, Nakatani E, Yagi H, Moriki M, Sano Y, Miyachi Y. Late-onset development of psoriasis in Japan: A population-based cohort study. JAAD International. 2021;**2**:51-61

[50] Frankel HC, Han J, Li T, Qureshi AA. The association between physical activity and the risk of incident psoriasis. Archives of Dermatology. 2012;**148**:918-924

[51] Queirós CS, Freitas JP. Sun exposure: Beyond the risks. Dermatology Practical & Conceptual. 31 Oct 2019;**9**(4):249-252. DOI: 10.5826/dpc.0904a01

[52] Karampinis E, Goudouras G, Ntavari N, Bogdanos DP, Roussaki-Schulze A-V, Zafiriou E. Serum vitamin D levels can be predictive of psoriasis flares up after COVID-19 vaccination: A retrospective case control study. Frontiers in Medicine (Lausanne). 2023;**10**

[53] Fowles J. Application of toxicological risk assessment principles to the chemical constituents of cigarette smoke. Tobacco Control. 2003;**12**:424-430

[54] Szentkereszty-Kovács Z, Gáspár K, Szegedi A, Kemény L, Kovács D, Törőcsik D. Alcohol in psoriasis—From bench to bedside. International Journal of Molecular Sciences. 2021;**22**:4987

[55] Csordas A, Bernhard D. The biology behind the atherothrombotic effects of cigarette smoke. Nature Reviews. Cardiology. 2013;**10**:219-230

[56] Armstrong AW, Harskamp CT, Dhillon JS, Armstrong EJ. Psoriasis and smoking: A systematic review and meta-analysis. British Journal of Dermatology. 2014;**170**:304-314

[57] Setty AR, Curhan G, Choi HK. Smoking and the risk of psoriasis in women: Nurses' health study II. The American Journal of Medicine. 2007;**120**:953-959

[58] Malakou LS, Gargalionis AN, Piperi C, Papadavid E, Papavassiliou AG, Basdra EK. Molecular mechanisms of mechanotransduction in psoriasis. Annals of Translational Medicine. 2018;**6**:245-245

[59] Grodner C, Beauchet A, Fougerousse A-C, Quiles-Tsimaratos N, Perrot J-L, Barthelemy H, et al. Tattoo complications in treated and non-treated psoriatic patients. Journal of the European Academy of Dermatology and Venereology. 2020;**34**:888-896

[60] Teng Y, Xie W, Tao X, Liu N, Yu Y, Huang Y, et al. Infection-provoked psoriasis: Induced or aggravated (review). Experimental and Therapeutic Medicine. 2021;**21**:567

[61] Zhou S, Yao Z. Roles of infection in psoriasis. International Journal of Molecular Sciences. 2022;**23**:6955

[62] Spaulding AR, Salgado-Pabón W, Kohler PL, Horswill AR, Leung DYM, Schlievert PM. Staphylococcal and streptococcal Superantigen exotoxins. Clinical Microbiology Reviews. 2013;**26**:422-447

[63] Baker B, Laman J, Powles A, van der Fits L, Voerman J, Melief M-J, et al. Peptidoglycan and peptidoglycan-specific Th1 cells in psoriatic skin lesions. The Journal of Pathology. 2006;**209**:174-181

[64] Azizzadeh M, Nejad ZV, Ghorbani R, Pahlevan D. Relationship

between *helicobacter pylori* infection and psoriasis. Annals of Saudi Medicine. 2014;**34**:241-244

[65] Hübner AM, Tenbaum SP. Complete remission of palmoplantar psoriasis through helicobacter pylori eradication: A case report. Clinical and Experimental Dermatology. 2008;**33**:339-340

[66] Imafuku S, Nakayama J. Profile of patients with psoriasis associated with hepatitis C virus infection. The Journal of Dermatology. 2013;**40**:428-433

[67] Karampinis E, Gravani A, Gidarokosta P, Bogdanos DP, Roussaki-Schulze A-V, Zafiriou E. Pustular eruption following COVID-19 vaccination: A narrative case-based review. Vaccines (Basel). 2023;**11**:1298

[68] Ozaras R, Berk A, Ucar DH, Duman H, Kaya F, Mutlu H. Covid-19 and exacerbation of psoriasis. Dermatologic Therapy. 2020;**33**(4):e13632. DOI: 10.1111/dth.13632

[69] Efanova E, Bushueva O, Saranyuk R, Surovtseva A, Churnosov M, Solodilova M, et al. Polymorphisms of the GCLC gene are novel genetic markers for susceptibility to psoriasis associated with alcohol abuse and cigarette smoking. Life. 2023;**13**:1316

Chapter 4

Psychosocial Burden and Psychological Interventions for Patients with Psoriasis

Nicole Natarelli, Aleena Boby, Shaliz Aflatooni and Amanda Krenitsky

Abstract

Characterized by pruritic, scaly plaques, psoriasis is an immune-mediated chronic cutaneous condition associated with a negative impact on quality of life. In addition, psoriatic patients exhibit a greater incidence of anxiety and depression compared to the general population. The relationship between psoriasis and mental health has been shown to be bidirectional with disease activity worsening psychological burden, and psychological burden conversely impacting disease activity. While few studies to our knowledge precisely delineate the proportion of psoriatic patients with untreated mental health concerns, literature suggests many patients are not receiving optimal or timely mental health treatment. As such, researchers have explored various psychotherapeutic interventions to increase the quality of life among patients, including traditional psychotherapy, cognitive behavioral therapy, and various alternative modalities. This chapter seeks to discuss the psychological burden of psoriasis, both in relation to psychological comorbidity and overall quality of life. In addition, this chapter seeks to review evidence for psychological interventions for patients with psoriasis. A greater understanding of the mental health outcomes of psoriatic patients and psychological interventions may better equip clinicians with the necessary tools to treat psoriatic patients holistically, addressing both the physical and mental burden of the disease.

Keywords: psoriasis, anxiety, depression, quality of life, mental health, psychotherapy, cognitive behavioral therapy

1. Introduction

Psoriasis is an immune-mediated chronic cutaneous condition characterized by pruritic, scaly plaques on the extensor surfaces of skin. Morphological forms of psoriasis include plaque, flexural, futtate, pustual,or erythrodermic psoriasis, affecting an estimated 60 million people globally [1]. In addition to cutaneous symptoms, the association between psoriasis and increased psychological burden has long been established. The early 20th century brought greater interest in investigating the relationship between psoriasis and psychological factors. In 1907, French dermatologist

François detailed his observation of reduced mental health among patients with psoriasis and hypothesized psychological factors may exacerbate psoriatic severity [2]. In the early 1920s, American dermatologist William H. Goeckerman studied the efficacy of his treatment approach, the Goeckerman regimen, and noted improvements in psoriatic patients' mental health alongside physical symptoms [3]. Similarly, John H. Ingram developed the Ingram regimen, and research detailing its associated psychological impact was published in the early 2000s [4]. Since then, various studies have explored associations between psoriasis and mental health, including psychological comorbidities, factors that increase the risk of psychological burden, the bidirectional relationship between mental health and psoriasis, and overall quality of life.

The bidirectional relationship between psoriasis and mental health describes a phenomenon in which psoriasis may increase psychological burden, while increased psychological burden may be a trigger for worsening psoriasis. Peripheral nervous system pathways, the hypothalamic-pituitary-adrenal axis, the sympathetic-adrenal-medullary system, and immune-mediated pathways collectively contribute to the relationship between psoriasis and physiological stress [5]. For example, while psoriasis may contribute to anxiety due to factors such as chronic pruritus, disfigurement, stigmatization, and reduced social support, anxiety can further contribute to psoriasis via stress disturbances in the epidermal barrier, increased stress-related neuropeptides within psoriatic plaques, dysregulation of the hypothalamus-pituitary-adrenal axes, upregulation of stress-induced mast cells, natural killer cells, and cutaneous lymphocyte-associated antigen, and increased dendritic epidermal serotonin transporter protein expression. Similarly, depression can mediate psoriatic symptoms via mechanisms such as modulating itch perception and increasing the levels of pro-inflammatory cytokines and substance P, which promotes keratinocyte proliferation, cutaneous inflammation, and lymphocyte activation [5]. Unaddressed mental health among psoriatic patients risks a vicious cycle in which disease state may worsen mental health status, which in turn can exacerbate psoriasis.

2. Psychological burden of psoriasis

2.1 Psoriasis and quality of life (QoL)

In addition to specific psychological comorbidities, studies have assessed the general association between psoriasis and quality of life. A 2004 systematic review of 17 studies found a reduced quality of life among psoriatic patients, owing to physical discomfort, impaired emotional functioning, a negative body and self-image, and limitations in daily activities [6]. Specifically, the authors found an overall mean Dermatology Life Quality Index (DLQI) of 23.4, Pain Disability Index (PDI) scores ranging from 16.5–44, Short Form-36 (SF-36) scores ranging from 41.2–55.5 (physical component) and 45.2–50.9 (mental component), and mean Sickness Impact Profile (SIP) scores ranging from 8.9 to 10.2. **Table 1** details the interpretation of these scores.

Furthermore, authors found that higher age was associated with slightly higher levels of psychological functioning and quality of life, albeit slightly lower levels of physical functioning [6].

Given potential differences in quality of life among psoriatic patients of different ages, a 2017 systematic review and meta-analysis including 17 studies and 1185 patients evaluated health-related quality of life (HRQOL) specifically among children and adolescents with psoriasis [7]. Results revealed a weighted mean Children's

QoL tool	Score interpretation
DLQI	DLQI score 0–1: no effect on QoL DLQI score 2–5: small effect on QoL DLQI score 6–10: moderate effect on QoL DLQI score 11–20: very large effect on QoL DLQI score 21–30: extremely large effect on QoL
PDI	Score range 0–45, with a higher score indicating greater QoL impairment
SF-36	Score range 0–100, with a lower score indicating greater QoL impairment
SIP	Score range 0–100, with a higher score indicating greater QoL impairment

Table 1.
Score interpretation for QoL tools.

Dermatology Life Quality Index (CDLQI)/DLQI score of 7.7 (95% CI: 6.67–8.73) among studies, albeit with large study heterogeneity. Similar to the DLQI, higher CDLQI scores indicate greater negative effects on QoL. Furthermore, study samples with a higher percentage of girls were associated with greater HRQOL. In contrast, a higher mean age of onset was associated with a lower HRQOL [7].

Similarly, a 2016 study analyzing QoL among children with various dermatologic conditions found an average CDLQI score of 8.0 among patients with psoriasis (95% Confidence Interval (CI): 3.9–12.1), with a range of 0–29 [8]. Of the other analyzed dermatologic conditions, only atopic eczema (score of 8.5 (7.1–9.8)) and scabies (score of 9.2 (0–20.3)) depicted greater average CDLQI scores. Conversely, CDLQI scores for patients with psoriasis were greater than average scores for acne, alopecia, molluscum contagiosum, urticaria, vitiligo, and warts, suggesting a greater impact on quality of life [8].

2.2 Psoriasis and psychological comorbidities

In addition to quality of life, numerous studies globally have evaluated the association between psoriasis and specific psychological comorbidities. A 2023 publication detailed global epidemiology trends of mental health comorbidity in patients with psoriasis from 1986 to 2019 using five databases [9]. 56 studies were analyzed, with a cumulative prevalence of depression, anxiety, and suicide among psoriatic adults of 20%, 21%, and 0.77%, respectively. Furthermore, the respective incidence of depression, anxiety, and suicide was 42.1, 24.7, and 2.6 per 1000 person-years. Interestingly, patients in North America demonstrated a higher relative prevalence of depression and suicide, whereas patients in South America demonstrated a higher relative prevalence of anxiety [9].

Similarly, a 2017 systematic review of 34 included studies evaluated the prevalence of mental health disorders in psoriasis [10]. The prevalence of psychiatric conditions ranged from 24–90% across studies. Cumulatively, sleep disorders were the most prevalent among patients at 62.0%. Sexual dysfunction (45.6%), personality disorders (35.0%), anxiety (30.4%), adjustment disorder (29.0%), depression (27.6%), and substance-related and addictive disorders (24.8%) were also described [10].

Lastly, a 2022 analysis including 24 studies found patients with psoriasis are 1.5 times more likely to depict depressive symptoms than the general population. In addition, anxiety symptoms (20–50%), schizophrenia (2.82%), and suicidal ideation (12.7%) were more prevalent among psoriatic patients [11]. **Table 2** summarizes the results of six systematic reviews that discuss psychological comorbidity and psoriasis.

Author (Year)	Studies included	Depression	Anxiety	Other
Dowlatshahi et al. [12]	98	Prevalence: • 28% via questionnaires • 12% via ICD codes • 19% via DSM IV • 9% with antidepressant use Odds: 1.57 (95% CI: 1.40–1.76)	N/A	N/A
Ferreira [10]	34	Prevalence: 27.6%	Prevalence: 30.4%	• Sleep disorder: 62.0% • Sexual dysfunction: 45.6% • Personality disorder: 35.0% • Adjustment disorder: 29.0% • Substance-related and addictive disorder: 24.8%
Lukmanji et al. [13]	17	Odds: 1.48 (95% CI: 1.16–1.89)	N/A	N/A
Jalenques et al. [14]	101	N/A	• Social anxiety disorder prevalence: 15% (95% CI: 9–21%) • Generalized anxiety disorder: 11% (95% CI: 9–14%) • Unspecified anxiety: 9% (95% CI: 8–10%) • Anxiety symptoms: 34% (95% CI: 32–37%) • Odds of anxiety symptoms: 2.51 (95% CI: 2.02 to 3.12)	N/A
Hedemann et al. [11]	24	Odds: 1.5	Prevalence: 20–50%	• Schizophrenia: 2.82% • Suicidal ideation: 2.7%
Liu et al. [9]	56	Prevalence (adults): 20%	Prevalence (adults): 21%	Suicide (adults): 0.77%

Abbreviations: CI, Confidence Interval; ICD, International Classification of Diseases; DSM IV, Diagnostic and Statistical Manual of Mental Disorders IV

Table 2.
Systematic reviews of psychological comorbidity and psoriasis.

2.3 Factors associated with increased psychological burden

While an association exists between psoriasis and depression, anxiety, and other mental health disorders, particular disease factors may increase the risk of psychological burden. One of the most widely discussed factors associated with worse quality of life outcomes is the severity of disease. An internet-based questionnaire study conducted in China including 497 patients with psoriasis found a greater proportion of patients with severe disease to have mental stress vs. those with mild to moderate disease (99.0% vs. 73.2%, $p < 0.01$) [15]. Furthermore, rates of suicidal ideation were greater among those with severe disease (46.3% vs. 14.2%, $p < 0.01$), in addition to the proportion of patients who had suicidal behavior (6.8% vs. 1.1%, $p < 0.01$). Similarly, a 2020 study on the impact of psoriasis on quality of life among 51 patients found higher Psoriasis Area and Severity Index (PASI) scores had a significant impact on the psychological aspect of quality of life ($r = 0.41$) [16]. A higher PASI score correlated with greater anxiety, both currently and in general, and depression ($r = 0.33$, $4 = 0.35$, $r = 0.35$). In addition to disease severity as measured by PASI, authors also found illness duration negatively correlated with subjective quality of life ($r = -0.29$) and positively correlated with anxiety and depression ($r = 044$, $r = 0.38$).

Lastly, the association between disease severity and psychological burden was illustrated in a systematic review including 13 randomized-controlled trials of biological agents for the treatment of moderate-to-severe psoriasis [17]. Authors found DLQI improvements were associated with percentage of PASI improvement from baseline; in other words, an improvement in psoriatic disease state was associated with an improvement in DLQI. Biological agents demonstrating the greatest DLQI improvement were those demonstrating >75% mean reduction in PASI. Lastly, all treatment arms that demonstrated a mean PASI reduction of at least 75% predicted a mean shift from DLQI band 3 ("very much") to DLQI band 1 ("a little" impact on QoL) [17]. Collectively, these studies suggest increased disease severity is associated with a greater impact on QoL.

In addition to disease severity and disease duration, other factors have been described in the literature. Pruritus, one of the most reportedly distressing symptoms of psoriasis, has been associated with worse depressive symptoms [18]. Furthermore, a 2004 survey-based study including 266 patients with psoriasis in the United States found that in addition to greater body surface area affected, patient youth, and female gender were significantly associated with greater reductions in quality of life [19]. As patient youth may increase the psychological burden of disease, a 2018 interview-based study was conducted to better understand the qualitative experience of adolescents with psoriasis [7]. In total, six main themes of psoriasis-related HRQoL were described, including "physical symptoms," "feeling different," "psoriasis-related worry about the future," "increased attention," "attempts to conceal skin," and "treatment-related frustrations and worry." Authors described many reported challenges arising from appearance-related concerns.

Lastly, a 2021 study evaluated the association between mental health status and the level of agreement between physician and patient ratings of psoriasis severity [20]. Of the 502 patients analyzed, 43 (9%) and 49 (10%) screened positive for depression and anxiety, respectively. Overall, patients rated their psoriasis as less severe during 26% of visits and more severe during 13% of visits compared with their physician. Yet, those with positive anxiety or depression screenings were more likely to rate their psoriasis as more severe than their physician (relative risk ratio: 2.7 for depression, 95% CI: 1.6–4.5; 2.1 for anxiety; 95% CI: 1.3–3.4). Thus, the authors concluded discordance between patient and physician psoriatic severity ratings is associated with anxiety or depression [20].

2.4 Proportion of psoriatic patients seeking care for mental health

While studies suggest many psoriatic patients are not receiving optimal or timely mental health treatment, few studies exist to our knowledge delineating the proportion of patients with untreated mental health concerns. Yet, a 2023 cross-sectional study in China evaluated psychological neglect among patients with various common skin diseases, including but not limited to psoriasis [21]. Among 1010 dermatologic patients participating in the survey, 273 (27.0%) patients demonstrated a need for mental health intervention despite a lack of treatment, fulfilling the "with need" criteria. Furthermore, the authors describe contributing factors including a lack of knowledge about the availability of mental health services, a lack of knowledge regarding where to retrieve help, and concerns about treatment side effects [21]. Similarly, an internet-based questionnaire study conducted in China with 497 patients with psoriasis found up to 88.9% of patients had untreated psychological concerns [15].

While untreated mental distress appears to be prevalent among patients with psoriasis, a 96.7% weighted consensus agreement was found among 18 European experts for the following statement: "Assessing the impact on the mental health status of patients should be one of the aims of any multidisciplinary approach to elevating standards of care for patients living with psoriasis" [22]. Increased incorporation of multidisciplinary care may offset the prevalence of untreated mental health concerns. In addition, mental health discussions and resources should be provided at the time of diagnosis to ensure patients are equipped with the necessary tools to seek support, whether or not there are signs of current psychological distress.

3. Evidence-based psychological interventions for psoriasis

3.1 Current treatment recommendations

Despite the high prevalence of psychiatric disorders in psoriasis patients, there remains a notable scarcity of evidence-based clinical guidelines to help physicians effectively address these mental health concerns. As depression and anxiety are the most common psychiatric comorbidities in individuals with psoriasis, universal screening for these conditions is strongly recommended [11]. The 9-item Patient Health Questionnaire (PHQ-9) and the 7-item Generalized Anxiety Disorder Scale (GAD-7) are two common questionnaires that clinicians can incorporate into their assessments [23].

For patients exhibiting severe psychiatric symptoms or signs of suicidal ideation, a referral for psychiatric consultation is essential [11]. In such cases, involving specialized mental health professionals is crucial to ensure appropriate and timely intervention. Conversely, patients with mild or moderate psychiatric symptoms may rely on recommendations from their primary healthcare team. Interestingly, treatments aimed at managing psoriatic symptoms can also have a positive impact on depressive symptoms [24]. In addition, biologic treatments are highly recommended due to their potential to alleviate symptoms of anxiety and depression independent of skin inflammation [25]. To address the complex interplay between dermatological and psychiatric disorders, there is a growing demand for increased access to psychodermatology services. Through this multidisciplinary approach, healthcare providers can work together to improve the overall well-being and outcomes of psoriasis patients experiencing mental health challenges.

3.2 Psychotherapy and cognitive behavioral therapy

Numerous studies have demonstrated the positive effects of cognitive behavioral therapy (CBT) and other types of psychotherapy in combination with traditional dermatological treatments for improving depression and anxiety symptoms among patients with psoriasis [26]. One such study, conducted by Fortune et al. (2002), examined various psychological parameters in psoriasis patients who participated in a 6-week CBT program with weekly individual sessions in addition to their standard treatment [27]. The results revealed that integrating CBT with psoriasis treatment led to a significant reduction in the clinical severity of psoriasis ($p = 0.0001$), anxiety ($p = 0.0001$), depression ($p = 0.0001$), and psoriasis-related stress ($p = 0.001$) at both 6 weeks and 6 months post-intervention [27]. Another study, conducted by Zachariae et al., investigated the impact of 7 individual psychotherapy sessions over 12 weeks on perceived stress, as measured by the Brief Stress Questionnaire [28]. The researchers found a significant reduction in perceived stress from baseline to post-intervention in the treatment group compared to the control group ($p < 0.05$) [28]. Moreover, within the treatment group, there were significant improvements in psoriasis activity measures, including PASI, Total Sign Score, and Laser Doppler Skin Blood Flow [28]. These findings collectively indicate that therapy, particularly CBT and other types of psychotherapy, may play a crucial role in improving both psychological well-being and psoriasis symptoms in patients. The integration of psychological interventions alongside traditional dermatological treatments presents a promising approach to addressing the multifaceted impact of psoriasis on patients' mental health and overall QoL. **Table 3** summarizes the results of the reported two studies evaluating psychotherapy or CBT among psoriasis patients, in addition to two additional studies demonstrating significant effects.

3.3 Alternative psychological interventions

In addition to psychotherapy, researchers have explored the effects of various other psychological interventions on psoriasis, including group psychoeducational training, telephone-based motivational interviewing, and emotional disclosure therapy. In a 2017 study, Singh et al. assessed the impact of three psychoeducational training sessions held every 2 weeks on the severity of psoriasis and psychological outcomes [31]. The authors reported significant improvements in PASI, DLQI, and WHO-5 well-being index, indicating the effectiveness of psychoeducational training in enhancing both disease severity and emotional well-being. In addition, a 2014 study by Larsen et al. investigated the effects of a 3-month motivational interviewing intervention following climate/heliotherapy in psoriasis patients [32]. Similar to Singh et al., these researchers also observed significant improvements in various measures, including Self-Administered Psoriasis Area and Severity Index scores, the three self-management domains of the Health Education Impact Questionnaire, self-efficacy scores, illness perception, and several lifestyle change parameters. These study findings highlight the potential of using motivational interviewing to not only enhance medical management but also improve mental well-being related to the disease. Lastly, a 2010 study by Paradisi et al. explored the impact of two different emotional writing disclosure interventions on psoriasis patients undergoing ultraviolet B therapy [33]. Patients were divided into the PW group, where they were instructed to write about stressful events, the KW group, where they were instructed to write about major life goals, and the control group. Although PASI scores improved significantly in all three groups, the PW group exhibited a significant improvement in Skindex-29 values compared to the other groups [33]. This suggests that writing or talking about tense life events can be therapeutic, improve mental health and potentially improve disease status. **Table 3** summarizes the results of the three studies evaluating alternative psychological interventions that have been explored and shown significant psychological effects.

3.4 Current research

As the field of psychodermatology gains momentum, there is a pressing need for more targeted research investigating these specific interventions. A comprehensive understanding of treatment options that can effectively enhance mental health outcomes for patients with psoriasis is necessary. In a 2020 analysis, researchers reviewed existing human clinical trials that assessed the effects of psychotherapy with major cognitive

Author (Year)	Treatment	Results
Zachariae et al. [28]	5 1.5 h individual psychotherapy sessions, in person	• Significant reduction in Psoriasis Area Severity Index, Total Sign Score, and Laser Doppler Skin Blood Flow within treatment group • No change within control group
Fortune et al. [27]	6 2.5 h group CBT sessions, in person	Significant reduction in the clinical severity of psoriasis ($p = 0.0001$), anxiety ($p = 0.0001$), depression ($p = 0.0001$), and psoriasis-related stress ($p = 0.001$) at both 6 weeks and 6 months post-intervention
Bundy et al. [29]	6 online self CBT modules	• Anxiety scores were significantly reduced ($p < 0.05$) • Depression scores did not change psoriasis severity scores did not change
Price et al. [30]	8 1.5 h group psychotherapy sessions, in person	• Levels of anxiety were significantly reduced • No significant difference in levels of depression •
Singh et al. [31]	3 multidisciplinary educational sessions, every 2 weeks, 30–45 min	• Significant improvements in PASI, DLQI, and WHO-5 well-being index
Larsen et al. [32]	6 motivational interviewing sessions within 3 months	• Significant improvements in various measures, including Self-Administered Psoriasis Area and Severity Index scores, the three self-management domains of the Health Education Impact Questionnaire, self-efficacy scores, illness perception, and several lifestyle change parameters
Paradisi et al. [33]	3 sessions of emotional disclosure therapy (KW or PW)	• PASI scores improved significantly in all three groups • The PW group exhibited a significant improvement in Skindex-29 values compared to the other groups

KW, King's emotional writing intervention; PW, Pennebaker's emotional writing intervention

Table 3.
Studies on various psychological interventions in psoriasis patients.

and behavioral components on both psoriatic and psychological symptoms. The studies encompassed diverse psychotherapy interventions, including mindfulness-based cognitive therapy and cognitive-behavioral symptom management programs [26]. Although all the studies examined psychotherapy interventions, the review highlighted the clear lack of standardization in methodology among each of the studies, leading to an inability to properly compare the studies and draw meaningful conclusions.

One notable area for improvement in future studies is the consideration of psychiatric diagnosis or symptoms during the screening process. Differing inclusion criteria across studies may influence the observed magnitude of change in psychological symptoms within each trial. Moreover, researchers should strive for greater diversity in the study population. A broader approach can lead to a better representation of the global psoriasis population and enhance the generalizability of the findings. In addition, to strengthen the reliability and validity of study outcomes, future research should incorporate more clinician-based ratings in addition to self-reported measures. Lastly, to determine the effects of psychological intervention in a controlled setting, future studies should consider requiring participants maintain a stable dermatologic regimen during their participation. A stable treatment regimen ensures that any observed changes in psychological symptoms can be more confidently attributed to psychotherapy interventions rather than fluctuations in dermatological management. By addressing these areas of improvement, future research can enhance our understanding of the interplay between psychotherapy, psoriasis, and mental health, and the findings will help guide the development of more targeted and effective interventions to improve the overall well-being of individuals living with psoriasis.

4. Conclusion

Characterized by pruritic, scaly plaques on extensor surfaces, psoriasis is an immune-mediated chronic cutaneous condition associated with a reduced quality of life and various psychological comorbidities. Research suggests the relationship between psoriasis and mental health is bidirectional; namely, psoriasis may increase psychological burden, as increased psychological burden may promote disease activity. Many psoriatic patients do not receive adequate mental health support, although researchers and clinicians alike have explored possible therapeutic strategies to foster greater quality of life among patients. Evidence exists for the efficacy of psychotherapy and cognitive behavioral therapy, both in person and online. Other assessed strategies include educational sessions, motivational interviewing sessions, and emotional disclosure therapy. Clinicians must remain aware of the potential psychological impacts of psoriatic disease in order to promptly intervene. A holistic approach is warranted for the management of psoriasis, with attention to both the physical and mental components of the disease.

Abbreviations

CDLQI	Children's Dermatology Life Quality Index
CI	Confidence Interval
DLQI	Dermatology Life Quality Index
DSM IV	Diagnostic and Statistical Manual of Mental Disorders IV
HRQOL	Health-Related Quality of Life

ICD	International Classification of Diseases
PASI	Psoriasis Area and Severity Index
PDI	Psoriasis Disability Index
QoL	Quality of Life
SF-36	Short Form-36
SIP	Sickness Impact Profile
CBT	cognitive behavioral therapy (CBT)
PW	Pennebaker's emotional writing intervention
KW	King's emotional writing intervention

Author details

Nicole Natarelli[1*], Aleena Boby[1], Shaliz Aflatooni[1] and Amanda Krenitsky[2]

1 University of South Florida, Morsani College of Medicine, Tampa, FL, USA

2 Department of Dermatology and Cutaneous Surgery, University of South Florida, Tampa, FL, USA

*Address all correspondence to: natarellin@usf.edu

References

[1] Raharja A, Mahil SK, Barker JN. Psoriasis: A brief overview. Clinical Medicine (London, England). 2021;**21**(3):170-173. DOI: 10.7861/clinmed.2021-0257

[2] Hallopeau FH. La psoriasis et la nervosité. Annales de Dermatologie et de Syphiligraphie. 1907;**8**:477-481

[3] Griffiths CEM, Clark CM, Chalmers RJG, et al. The psychological effects of Goeckerman treatment for psoriasis. The British Journal of Dermatology. 1989;**121**(6):751-757

[4] Fortune DG, Richards HL, Griffiths CE, et al. The psychological impact of an Ingram regimen outpatient treatment on patients with psoriasis. The British Journal of Dermatology. 2002;**147**(1):193-200

[5] Ferreira BIRC, Abreu JLPDC, Reis JPGD, Figueiredo AMDC. Psoriasis and associated psychiatric disorders. The Journal of Clinical and Aesthetic Dermatology. 2016;**9**(6):36-43

[6] de Korte J, Sprangers MA, Mombers FM, Bos JD. Quality of life in patients with psoriasis: A systematic literature review. The Journal of Investigative Dermatology: Symposium Proceedings. 2004;**9**(2):140-147. DOI: 10.1046/j.1087-0024.2003.09110.x

[7] Randa H, Todberg T, Skov L, Larsen LS, Zachariae R. Health-related quality of life in children and adolescents with psoriasis: A systematic review and meta-analysis. Acta Dermato-Venereologica. 2017;**97**(5):555-563. DOI: 10.2340/00015555-2600

[8] Olsen JR, Gallacher J, Finlay AY, Piguet V, Francis NA. Quality of life impact of childhood skin conditions measured using the Children's Dermatology Life Quality Index (CDLQI): A meta-analysis. The British Journal of Dermatology. 2016;**174**(4):853-861. DOI: 10.1111/bjd.14361

[9] Liu L, Lin NX, Yu YT, et al. Epidemiology of mental health comorbidity in patients with psoriasis: An analysis of trends from 1986 to 2019. Psychiatry Research. 2023;**321**:115078. DOI: 10.1016/j.psychres.2023.115078

[10] Ferreira BR, Pio-Abreu JL, Reis JP, Figueiredo A. Analysis of the prevalence of mental disorders in psoriasis: The relevance of psychiatric assessment in dermatology. Psychiatria Danubina. 2017;**29**(4):401-406. DOI: 10.24869/psyd.2017.401

[11] Hedemann TL, Liu X, Kang CN, Husain MI. Associations between psoriasis and mental illness: An update for clinicians. General Hospital Psychiatry. 2022;**75**:30-37. DOI: 10.1016/j.genhosppsych.2022.01.006

[12] Dowlatshahi EA, Wakkee M, Arends LR, Nijsten T. The prevalence and odds of depressive symptoms and clinical depression in psoriasis patients: A systematic review and meta-analysis. The Journal of Investigative Dermatology. 2014;**134**(6):1542-1551. DOI: 10.1038/jid.2013.508

[13] Lukmanji A, Basmadjian RB, Vallerand IA, Patten SB, Tang KL. Risk of depression in patients with psoriatic disease: A systematic review and meta-analysis. Journal of Cutaneous Medicine and Surgery. 2021;**25**(3):257-270. DOI: 10.1177/1203475420977477

[14] Jalenques I, Bourlot F, Martinez E, et al. Prevalence and odds of anxiety

disorders and anxiety symptoms in children and adults with psoriasis: Systematic review and meta-analysis. Acta Dermato-Venereologica. 2022;**102**:adv00769. DOI: 10.2340/actadv.v102.1386

[15] Xiaolan C, Liying Z, Hao Z, Jianzhong Z, Zhang Chunlei J, Jun MG, et al. Disease burden and quality of life in patients with psoriasis: An internet-based questionnaire. Chinese Journal of Dermatology. 2019;**52**(11):791-795

[16] Bulat V, Šitum M, Delaš Aždajić M, Lovrić I, Dediol I. Study on the impact of psoriasis on quality of life: Psychological, social and financial implications. Psychiatria Danubina. 2020;**32**(Suppl. 4):553-561

[17] Mattei PL, Corey KC, Kimball AB. Psoriasis Area Severity Index (PASI) and the Dermatology Life Quality Index (DLQI): The correlation between disease severity and psychological burden in patients treated with biological therapies. Journal of the European Academy of Dermatology and Venereology. 2014;**28**(3):333-337. DOI: 10.1111/jdv.12106

[18] Gupta MA, Pur DR, Vujcic B, Gupta AK. Suicidal behaviors in the dermatology patient. Clinics in Dermatology. 2017;**35**(3):302-311. DOI: 10.1016/j.clindermatol.2017.01.006

[19] Gelfand JM, Feldman SR, Stern RS, Thomas J, Rolstad T, Margolis DJ. Determinants of quality of life in patients with psoriasis: A study from the US population. Journal of the American Academy of Dermatology. 2004;**51**(5):704-708. DOI: 10.1016/j.jaad.2004.04.014

[20] Carr E, Mahil SK, Brailean A, et al. Association of patient mental health status with the level of agreement between patient and physician ratings of psoriasis severity. JAMA Dermatology. 2021;**157**(4):413-420. DOI: 10.1001/jamadermatol.2020.5844

[21] Tang TR, Wang M, Li H, et al. Untreated depression and anxiety in patients with common skin diseases: A cross-sectional study in China. Frontiers in Psychology. 2023;**14**:1150998. DOI: 10.3389/fpsyg.2023.1150998

[22] Koren J, Lambert JLW, Thomsen SF, et al. Elevating the standard of care for patients with psoriasis: "Calls to Action" from epicensus, a multistakeholder Pan-European initiative. Dermatologic Therapy. 2023;**13**(1):245-268. DOI: 10.1007/s13555-022-00846-3

[23] Kroenke K, Spitzer RL, Williams JBW, Löwe B. The patient health questionnaire somatic, anxiety, and depressive symptom scales: A systematic review. General Hospital Psychiatry. 2010;**32**(4):345-359. DOI: 10.1016/j.genhosppsych.2010.03.006

[24] Roubille C, Richer V, Starnino T, et al. Evidence-based recommendations for the management of comorbidities in rheumatoid arthritis, psoriasis, and psoriatic arthritis: Expert opinion of the canadian dermatology-rheumatology comorbidity initiative. The Journal of Rheumatology. 2015;**42**(10):1767-1780. DOI: 10.3899/jrheum.141112

[25] Fleming P, Bai JW, Pratt M, Sibbald C, Lynde C, Gulliver WP. The prevalence of anxiety in patients with psoriasis: A systematic review of observational studies and clinical trials. Journal of the European Academy of Dermatology and Venereology. 2017;**31**(5):798-807. DOI: 10.1111/jdv.13891

[26] Sijercic I, Ennis N, Monson CM. A systematic review of cognitive and

behavioral treatments for individuals with psoriasis. Journal of Dermatological Treatment. 2020;**31**(6):631-638. DOI: 10.1080/09546634.2019.1690625

[27] Fortune DG, Richards HL, Kirby B, Bowcock S, Main CJ, Griffiths CEM. A cognitive-behavioural symptom management programme as an adjunct in psoriasis therapy. The British Journal of Dermatology. 2002;**146**(3):458-465. DOI: 10.1046/j.1365-2133.2002.04622.x

[28] Zachariae R, Øster H, Bjerring P, Kragballe K. Effects of psychologic intervention on psoriasis: A preliminary report. Journal of the American Academy of Dermatology. 1996;**34**(6):1008-1015. DOI: 10.1016/S0190-9622(96)90280-7

[29] Bundy C, Pinder B, Bucci S, Reeves D, Griffiths CEM, Tarrier N. A novel, web-based, psychological intervention for people with psoriasis: The electronic Targeted Intervention for Psoriasis (eTIPs) study. The British Journal of Dermatology. 2013;**169**(2):329-336. DOI: 10.1111/bjd.12350

[30] Price ML, Mottahedin I, Mayo PR. Can psychotherapy help patients with psoriasis? Clinical and Experimental Dermatology. 1991;**16**(2):114-117. DOI: 10.1111/j.1365-2230.1991.tb00319.x

[31] Singh S, Narang T, Vinay K, et al. Clinic-based group multi-professional education causes significant decline in psoriasis severity: A randomized open label pilot study. Indian Dermatology Online Journal. 2017;**8**(6):454. DOI: 10.4103/idoj.IDOJ_68_17

[32] Larsen MH, Krogstad AL, Aas E, Moum T, Wahl AK. A telephone-based motivational interviewing intervention has positive effects on psoriasis severity and self-management: A randomized controlled trial. The British Journal of Dermatology. 2014;**171**(6):1458-1469. DOI: 10.1111/bjd.13363

[33] Paradisi A, Abeni D, Finore E, et al. Effect of written emotional disclosure interventions in persons with psoriasis undergoing narrow band ultraviolet B phototherapy. European Journal of Dermatology EJD. 2010;**20**(5):599-605. DOI: 10.1684/ejd.2010.1018

Section 3

Daring New Roads

Chapter 5

Biologics: Beyond the Basics

Ariel T. Kidron, Anthony P. Gulotta and Michael F. Land

Abstract

Biologics are novel targeted therapies aimed at blocking specific cells or proteins created by the immune system that mediate the inflammatory process. Currently, the American Food and Drug Administration (FDA) has approved 12 different biologics that are administered either through intravenous infusion or intramuscularly for the treatment and prevention of psoriasis and arthritic psoriasis. These biologics categorically inhibit different cytokines, mainly IL-23, IL-17A, and IL-17F, that are activated and mediate the psoriasiform process with better long-term effectiveness and reduced side effects as compared to traditional systemic and topical steroids. The benefit of biologics also extends to a larger time interval between medication dosing as patients may achieve therapeutic levels for weeks to months before needing another dose. Transition to biologics from standard therapy should be considered for the right patients who have failed to improve, however with caution towards inherently immunocompromised patients as biologics may increase the risk of developing infections through compounded immune system suppression. This risk can be stratified with prophylactic blood tests, TB testing, and other examinations while on the biologics to ensure proper patient safety and therapeutic benefit.

Keywords: psoriasis, biologics, immunology, pharmacology, dermatopathology

1. Introduction

Biologics are a different class of medications than traditional systemic drugs that target the entire immune system. These agents are able to specifically target parts of the immune system that may mediate a certain pathology without affecting other normal functioning aspects of the immune system and thus yield less risk of side effects involving the liver, kidneys and other organs typically affected by immunosuppressive medications [1]. The biologics used to treat psoriasis distinctively block a set of cytokines which are proteins that facilitate the immune system response. Cytokines such as tumor necrosis factor-alpha (TNF-alpha), interleukin 17-A, interleukin 12, and interleukin 23 serve a major role in manifesting the disease process of psoriasis and psoriatic arthritis which include joint damage, osteopenia, and chronic inflammation involving the skin and other organs [2, 3]. Currently there are 11 biologics that have been approved by the American FDA to treat psoriasis and arthritic psoriasis for both adults and children over 4 years of age [1, 3]. These approved biologics have a relatively good safety profile, however judicious discretion is warranted in selecting appropriate therapy for the right patient in order to achieve the best therapeutic outcome [1, 3].

2. TNF-a inhibitors

The adoption of biologic therapy has significantly enhanced the treatment of moderate to severe psoriasis. Earlier first line therapy was limited to oral agents such as methotrexate, cyclosporine and retinoids with extensive black box warnings and potential risk of death [3]. This advancement in therapy is linked to better understanding of the underlying pathophysiology of psoriasis as more extensive than hyperproliferation of the epidermis as previously postulated [3]. Recent literature has been able to produce a clear pathophysiological mechanism with direct association of specific cytokines in the disease process. In the first part of the pathophysiological cascade interleukin 12 and interleukin 23 are secreted from macrophages, keratinocytes, and natural killer T cells. These interleukins illicit the differentiation of native T cells to Th1, Th17, and Th22 cells which go on to produce tumor necrosis factor alpha (TNF-a), interleukin 17, and interleukin 22 which represent the ending inflammatory cascade [3–5]. The interleukin 23 mediated Th17 activation pathway has been identified as the major patho-immunological contributor in the inflammatory response involving psoriasis [3]. Current evidence shows that biologic treatment aimed at inhibiting TNF-a, interleukin 23, and Interleukin 17 has been more effective in treating psoriasis which further reinforces their greater roles in the disease process [5].

As the therapeutic apparatus enlarges and more treatment options become available the choice of which agent is more appropriate for which patient becomes harder to make. As a result, the use of biologics in the treatment of psoriasis can become both an art and a science. The earliest approved biologic option, Adalimumab (Humira), is a human monoclonal antibody targeting TNF-a and has been widely effective in reducing joint destruction in psoriatic arthritis patients and has been prescribed for plaque psoriasis in children [6]. An ongoing 10-year international prospective observational registry evaluating the long-term safety and effectiveness of adalimumab has shown low numbers of events adverse events including serious infections, cardiovascular pathology, or malignancy [7]. Data from the pregnancy inflammatory bowel disease and neonatal outcomes (PIANO) has also shown no increased risk of poor outcomes during pregnancy [8]. However, over prolonged use adalimumab has shown reduced efficacy as opposed to newer agents, in addition there is well documented and established association between TNF-a inhibitors and reactivation of the tuberculosis virus which mandates careful monitoring preinitiation of treatment [5].

Etanercept (Enbrel) is another a TNF-a inhibitor that is used for treatment of moderate to severe adult and pediatric plaque psoriasis as well as psoriatic arthritis, however, the use of this biologic has significantly decreased over the last 10 years due to its association with progressive multifocal leukoencephalopathy triggered by the human polyomavirus 2 [9]. Despite this association, Etanercept has been effectively utilized in the geriatric population as one of the best safety profile biologics in treatment of severe psoriasis and was the first biologic approved for pediatric use down to 4 years of age [5].

Infliximab (Remicade) is a TNF-a inhibitor approved for use in treatment of psoriasis, psoriatic arthritis and other inflammatory syndromes in both adults and children, however since it is administered intravenously it is not commonly utilized by dermatologists [5].

Certolizumab (Cimzia) is a TNF-a blocker that functions in a dose dependent manner. This biologic is utilized in the treatment of psoriatic arthritis and moderate to severe plaque psoriasis [5]. Certolizumab has maintained its efficacy in treatment of psoriatic arthritis in patients with and without prior use of other TNF-a inhibitors [10]. Certolizumab has shown superior efficacy in phase 3 clinical trials as compared with other TNF-a inhibitors, achieving a 75% improvement in the psoriasis area and severity index (PASI) in 81.6% of patients by week 16 since onset of first dose [11]. In addition, certolizumab has been demonstrated to be safe during pregnancy with minimal transfer across the placenta as well as into breast milk [12, 13]. Safety wise, certolizumab has recorded data only up to 3 years of use and it requires more frequent dosing than other biologics [5].

3. Interleukin-17 inhibitors

The subsequent class of biologic agents to be approved by the FDA focused their action on inhibiting interleukin-17A and the first biologic approved for plaque psoriasis and psoriatic arthritis in that class was secukinumab (Cosentyx). This agent has shown excellent efficacy in treating traditionally resistant disease domains including the scalp, nails, and palmoplantar psoriasis [14–16]. Furthermore, in a trial comparing secukinumab to etanercept and ustekinumab (interleukin-12/23 inhibitor), secukinumab showed superior results in clearing the skin of patients with moderate to severe plaque psoriasis [17]. Moreover, the American FDA has recognized secukinumab's efficacy in inhibiting joint destruction in patients with psoriatic arthritis and as a result it is currently the preferred agent for psoriatic arthritis as opposed to interleukin-12/23 or interleukin-23 inhibiting agents [18]. Secukinumab has also displayed significant recapturing properties, exhibiting a 75% improvement in PASI by week 12 in 95% of patients who discontinued and restarted the medication after experiencing a disease exacerbation [5]. There is an increased risk of new onset or exacerbation of existing inflammatory bowel disease with interleukin-17 inhibitors as well as minor risk of fungal and yeast infections [5]. Yet, secukinumab has no black box warnings issued by the American FDA and has been monitored the longest for safety out of all the interleukin-17 inhibitors [5, 19]. According to phase 3 clinical trials, while on secukinumab, fungal and yeast infection rates were higher than placebo but less than 1% and 1.3% respectively [5]. The incidence of new onset inflammatory bowel disease in patients taking secukinumab has been documented to be 0.001% of patients [5].

Brodalumab (Siliq) was the subsequent interleukin-17 inhibitor to be approved by the American FDA for the treatment of moderate to severe plaque psoriasis in adult patients [5]. Brodalumab's mechanism of action is unique among its class because it is the only biologic to completely inhibit all parts of the interleukin-17 receptor including 17A, 17F, 17A/F, and 17E [5]. As a result, brodalumab has shown excellent efficacy and rapid onset of action in phase 3 clinical trials accomplishing 100% improvement in the psoriasis area and severity index in 44% of patients by week 12 and since onset of first dose [5]. In comparison to ustekinumab, brodalumab's rapid onset of action achieved a statistically significant 90% improvement in the psoriasis area and severity index by 2 and 100% improvement by week 4 [5]. Additionally, brodalumab has shown effectiveness in rescuing patients from other failed and non-responsive interleukin-17A inhibitor treatment [20]. This effectiveness is compounded in literature displaying that by 52 weeks of treatment, less than 3% of patients developed resistance to treatment [5]. The American FDA has issued a warning for suicide regarding brodalumab, however no scientific evidence has emerged to show any increased risk of completed suicides, suicide attempts, major cardiac events, tuberculosis, or other inflammatory bowel diseases based on a recently published one-year pharmacovigilance study in 2020 [21]. In addition, analysis of the phase III clinical trials done around the world has shown 4 completed suicides in 4464 patients with all patients having an underlying or associated psychiatric disorders or stressors. Moreover, no other country except the United States has issued an increased risk of suicides with use of brodalumab [5, 22]. The incidence of new onset inflammatory bowel disease in patients taking brodalumab has been reported as 1 out of 4464 patients with the risk of yeast infection being 0.9% as opposed to 0.2% while on placebo [5]. Based upon the reassuring PASI data, cost effectiveness, as well as relatively safe profile, brodalumab serves as a first line treatment for moderate to severe psoriasis.

Ixekizumab (Talz) is another agent that inhibits the interleukin-17 receptor through blocking its interaction with the interleukin-17A receptor component [5]. This biologic is indicated for plaque psoriasis in adults and kids as early as 6 years of age, and it is the only American FDA approved actor for treatment of genital plaque psoriasis [5]. Ixekizumab has displayed superior effectiveness in treating moderate to severe pediatric plaque psoriasis during clinical trials as compared to placebo with similar safety profile results seen in adults [23]. Ixekizumab has shown a 75% improvement on the PASI scale in 90% patients by week 12 and has demonstrated superior results in onset of action and nail clearing when compared to other biologics such as adalimumab and guselkumab (interleukin-23 inhibitor) [24, 25]. Currently ixekizumab has no black box warning issued by the American FDA and has displayed a relatively safe profile of use with the incidence of inflammatory bowel disease development being less than 1 out of 1000 patients [5]. Like other interleukin-17 inhibitors, ixekizumab carries an increased risk of fungal and yeast infections however in phase 3 clinical trials the incidence of yeast infection was 0.6% as compared to 0.5% while on placebo [26].

Bimekizumab (Bimzelx) is a dual interleukin-17A and interleukin-17F inhibitor which has shown improved therapeutic benefit as compared to sole blockage of interleukin-17A and has been indicated for treatment of moderate to severe plaque psoriasis and psoriatic arthritis in adults [27]. In a head-to-head comparison, Bimekizumab has demonstrated better clinical results than ustekinumab (interleukin-12/23 inhibitor) that translated into achieving a 90% improvement in the PASI scale for 85% of patients by week 16 vs. 49.7% of patients on ustekinumab [28]. Furthermore, following one dose, bimekizumab has demonstrated quicker onset of response when compared with ustekinumab where, a 75% improvement on the PASI was observed in 76.9% of patients taking bimekizumab vs. 15.3% of the patients on ustekinumab [28]. Unfortunately, bimekizumab is still undergoing the approval process by the American FDA for use in plaque psoriasis and it is currently available throughout the European Union, Australia, and Asia.

4. Interleukin-23 inhibitors

The interleukin-23 inhibitors are a relatively newer class of biologic agents developed to treat plaque psoriasis and the first biologic in this class to be approved by the American FDA was guselkumab (Tremfya) [5]. This agent halts the immune cascade mediated through the interleukin-23 receptor by inhibiting the p19 subunit of the interleukin-23 receptor and is currently the only interleukin-23 inhibitor to also be approved for treatment of psoriatic arthritis [5]. Guselkumab has displayed excellent clinical results with achieving a 75% improvement on the PASI scale in 90% of patients by week 16 [29]. In a head-to-head comparison, guselkumab has shown superior clinical results against secukinumab in achieving a 90% improvement on the PASI scale at week 48, in addition to performing better than adalimumab in the treatment of scalp plaque psoriasis and palmoplantar psoriasis [30, 31]. Guselkumab reports a slower onset time when compared to ixekizumab, however, was able to achieve a similar end point by week 24 [5]. Safety wise, the drug has garnered safety data for over 3 years with no significant evidence for increased risk of tuberculosis, fungal infections, yeast infections, or inflammatory bowel disease [5].

Tildrakizumab (Ilumya) was the next interleukin-23 inhibitor to be approved by the American FDA and it functions through the same mechanism as its predecessor guselkumab by binding the p19 subunit of the interleukin-23 receptor and preventing its downstream participation in the immune cascade [5]. This drug is currently only approved for treatment of moderate to severe plaque psoriasis and has shown high recapture rates where approximately 85–96% of patients showed a 75% improvement on the PASI scale after stopping and restarting the medication [32]. Moreover, tildrakizumab has also demonstrated a sustained therapeutic effect without redosing, where patients were able to maintain a 75% improvement on the PASI scale for 7.4 months before losing their response [33]. Safety wise, tildrakizumab had least number of adverse effects occurring at least in 1% of patients among all the biologics available for treatment of psoriasis [5]. The downside to this biologic is that both the onset of action and peak efficacy are slower in comparison to other interleukin-23 inhibitors [5].

Risankizumab (Skyrizi) is the latest interleukin-23 inhibitor approved by American FDA and it exerts its antagonism of interleukin-23 by selectively targeting the p19 subunit of the interleukin-23 receptor [5]. The drug is currently indicated for moderate to severe plaque psoriasis in adults. Currently the drug requires four sets of dosing per year and one set of dosing per year is currently being reviewed by the American FDA [5]. Risankizumab has shown good efficacy in clinical trials with a 90% improvement on the PASI scale in 74.8%–75.3% of the patients by week 1 [5]. Risankizumab has also performed well in head-to-head trials, displaying superior efficacy in comparison to adalimumab, ustekinumab, and secukinumab with a similar fast onset as secukinumab [34–36]. Furthermore, risankizumab has shown high durability as patients experienced recurrence of moderate to severe pathology an average of 295 days post discontinuation [5]. Unfortunately, there is no long-term safety data available like older medications, however risankizumab has shown excellent safety profile data both for short term use (16 weeks) and for long term use including up to 69 months [37]. Like other interleukin-23 class agents, risankizumab has no concern for increased risk of inflammatory bowel disease or tuberculosis reactivation, and the most common adverse effects are upper respiratory infections, headache, and injection site infections [5].

Mirikizumab is the latest investigational interleukin-23 inhibitor which also targets the p19 subunit of the cytokine receptor however it is not yet approved by the American FDA for treatment of plaque psoriasis [5]. Clinical trial data has shown mirikizumab increases PASI by 90% by week 16 in 67% of the patients with the most common adverse effects being viral and upper respiratory tract infections [38]. Trials have also demonstrated that continued use for patients who do not achieve the primary end point of 90% improve in PASI scale by 16 weeks may achieve it with continued use up to 104 weeks [39].

5. Interleukin-12/23 inhibitors

The interleukin-12/23 inhibitors treat psoriasis by exhibiting a combination of blockade on the interleukin-12 and interleukin-23 receptors. Currently, ustekinumab (Stelara) is the only medication in this class that is FDA approved to treat moderate to severe plaque psoriasis and psoriatic arthritis in adults and pediatric population down to 6 years of age [5]. Ustekinumab's mechanism of action entails binding with high affinity and specificity to the p40 subunit of both the interleukin-12 and interleukin-23 receptors and suppressing the inflammation facilitated by these cytokines [40]. This agent is less efficacious than other biologics and some patients may experience worsening of psoriatic symptoms during the 3rd month of medication use and may benefit from an increased dose or an increased frequency of dosing [5]. Ustekinumab has long track record of good safety profile data for over 20 years and uniquely it is the only biologic approved for dose changes based on a patient's weight without increase risk of adverse events [5].

6. Conclusion

The arsenal of biologic options for the treatment of psoriasis is continually expanding with each agent containing its own merits and demerits with respect to other available biologics. After reviewing the facts of each biologic an informed clinician may cater the most appropriate therapy for the right patient so as to produce the best possible patient care and patient satisfaction (**Figure 1** and **Table 1**).

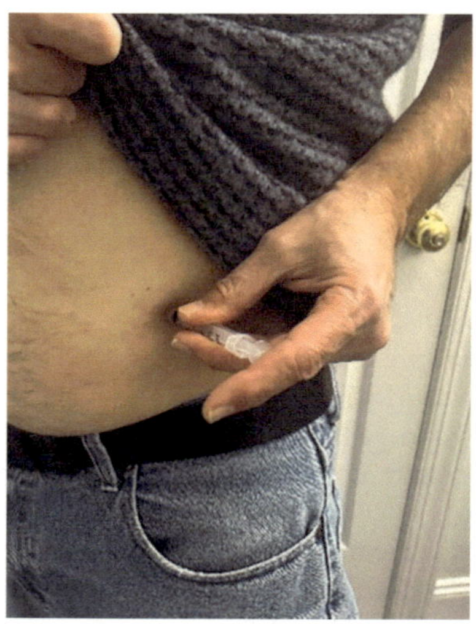

Figure 1.
Biologics are large molecule proteins that must be administered subcutaneously or intravenously. Subcutaneous injections can be delivered in multiple anatomical locations such as the outer surface of the upper arm, top of the thigh, the buttocks, or in the abdomen. In the photograph here, a patient self-administers a biologic treatment in the outer abdomen. Importantly, the abdominal injections must occur above the waistline and not include the navel.

DOI: http://dx.doi.org/10.5772/intechopen.1004056

Medication name (Brand Name)	Biologics class	Efficacy	Potential side effects	Average cost per month (US Dollars)
Infliximab (Remicade)	TNF-a Inhibitor	A 75% improvement from baseline PASI score in chronic recalcitrant plaque psoriasis by week 10. FDA indications for moderate to severe plaque psoriasis. Off label uses for pyoderma gangrenosum, hidradenitis suppurative, and Uveitis in Behcet's syndrome	Injection site reaction, headache, and rash. Also risk of serious infection, in particular, reactivation of latent tuberculosis. Evidence of infliximab-induced severe depression and suicide ideation	$987
Certolizumab (Cimzia)	TNF-a Inhibitor	Superior efficacy in phase 3 clinical trials as compared with other TNF-a inhibitors, achieving a 75% improvement in 81.6% of patients by week 16	Injection site reaction, headache, and rash. Also risk of serious infection, in particular, reactivation of latent tuberculosis. Evidence of optic neuritis, in ~3 patients out of 1000	$1, 040
Adalimumab (Humira)	TNF-a Inhibitor	78% of treated patients achieved 75% improvement at week 16	Injection site reaction, headache, and rash. Also risk of serious infection, in particular, reactivation of latent tuberculosis	$7, 000
Etanercept (Enbrel)	TNF-a Inhibitor	A 56% of patients achieving PASI 75 and 77% of patients achieving PASI 50 by week 24	Injection site reaction, headache, and rash. Also risk of serious infection, in particular, reactivation of latent tuberculosis	$10, 500
Bimekizumab (Bimzelx)	Interleukin-17 Inhibitor	A 90% improvement for 85% of patients by week 16 vs. 49.7% of patients on ustekinumab	Injection site reaction, headache, pimples (acne), nausea, and generalized fatigue	$2, 552
Brodalumab (Siliq)	Interleukin-17 Inhibitor	A 100% improvement in the psoriasis area and severity index in 44% of patients by week 12 and since onset of first dose	Injection site reaction, black tarry stools, headache, joint pain, nausea, and pale skin. American FDA warning for suicide ideation	$3, 500
Ixekizumab (Taltz)	Interleukin-17 Inhibitor	A 75% improvement in 90% of patients by week 12	Injection site reaction, arthralgias, headache, neutropenia, thrombocytopenia, and risk of candidiasis or tinea infections. Evidence of inflammatory bowel disease exacerbation, in less than 1 patient out of 1000	$6, 586
Secukinumab (Cosentyx)	Interleukin-17 Inhibitor	A 75% improvement in PASI by week 12 in 95% of patients who discontinued and restarted the medication after experiencing a disease exacerbation	Injection site reaction, inflammatory bowel disease flareups, arthralgias, back pain, cough, headache, pruritus, and rhinorrhea. Evidence of fungal and yeast infections, in ~12 patients out of 1000	$6, 924

Medication name (Brand Name)	Biologics class	Efficacy	Potential side effects	Average cost per month (US Dollars)
Guselkumab (Tremfya)	Interleukin-23 Inhibitor	A 75% improvement for 90% of patients by week 16. Shown superior clinical results against secukinumab in achieving a 90% improvement on the PASI scale at week 48, in addition to performing better than adalimumab in the treatment of scalp plaque psoriasis and palmoplantar psoriasis	Injection site reaction, arthralgias, diarrhea, headaches	\$1, 651
Mirikizumab (Omvoh)	Interleukin-23 Inhibitor	A 90% improvement by week 16 in 67% of patients	Arthralgias, headaches, viral and upper respiratory tract infections	\$9, 976
Tildrakizumab (Ilumya)	Interleukin-23 Inhibitor	Recapture rate where approximately 85–96% of patients showed a 75% improvement after stopping and starting medication in 85–96% of patients	Injection site reaction, diarrhea, and upper respiratory infections.	\$17, 296
Risankizumab (Skyrizi)	Interleukin-23 Inhibitor	A 90% improvement in 74.8%–75.3% of patients by week 1. Displaying superior efficacy in comparison to adalimumab, ustekinumab, and secukinumab with a similar fast onset as secukinumab	Headaches, swelling of face, eyelids, lips, mouth, tongue, or throat, hives or pruritus. May induce low blood pressure leading to dizziness, lightheadedness, and fainting. May cause burning with urination or increase urinary frequency	\$19, 734
Ustekinumab (Stelara)	Interleukin-12/23 Inhibitor	A 90% improvement by week 16 in 49.7% of patients	Injection site reaction, abdominal pain, diarrhea, headache, and generalized fatigue	\$2, 051

**Injection site reactions can include erythema, itching, pain, and swelling and usually last 1–3 days [41].*

Table 1.
Detailed synopsis of the biologics with appropriate indications, contraindications and comparisons amongst different classes.

Additional information

The views expressed herein are those of the authors and do not reflect the official policy or position of Brooke Army Medical Center, the U.S. Army Medical Department, the U.S. Army Office of the Surgeon General, the Department of the Army, the Department of the Air Force and Department of Defense or the U.S. Government.

Author details

Ariel T. Kidron[1]*, Anthony P. Gulotta[2] and Michael F. Land[1]

1 San Antonio Uniformed Services Health Education Consortium, San Antonio, Texas, United States

2 Walter Reed National Military Medical Center, Bethesda, Maryland, United States

*Address all correspondence to: dr.arielkidron@gmail.com

References

[1] Psoriasis treatment: Biologics. American Academy of Dermatology. 2022. Available from: https://www.aad.org/public/diseases/psoriasis/treatment/medications/biologics

[2] Tsai YC, Tsai TF. Anti-interleukin and interleukin therapies for psoriasis: Current evidence and clinical usefulness. Theraputic Advances in Musculoskeletal Disease. 2017;**9**(11):277-294. DOI: 10.1177/1759720X17735756

[3] Brownstone ND, Hong J, Mosca M, et al. Biologic treatments of psoriasis: An update for the clinician. Biologics. 2021;**15**:39-51. DOI: 10.2147/BTT.S252578

[4] Armstrong AW, Read C. Pathophysiology, clinical presentation, and treatment of psoriasis: A review. Journal of the American Medical Association. 2020;**323**(19):1945-1960. DOI: 10.1001/jama.2020.4006

[5] Alwan W, Nestle FO. Pathogenesis and treatment of psoriasis: Exploiting pathophysiological pathways for precision medicine. Clinical and Experimental Rheumatology. 2015;**33**(5 Suppl 93):S2-S6

[6] Elewski BE, Baker CS, Crowley JJ, et al. Adalimumab for nail psoriasis: Efficacy and safety over 52 weeks from a phase-3, randomized, placebo-controlled trial. Journal of the European Academy of Dermatology and Venereology. 2019;**33**(11):2168-2178. DOI: 10.1111/jdv.15793

[7] Wu JJ, Abramovits W, Valdecantos WC, et al. 10-year interim results from the ESPRIT registry: Real-world safety, effectiveness, and patient-reported outcomes of adalimumab for moderate-to-severe psoriasis. Journal of the American Academy of Dermatology. 2020;**83**(6):AB17. DOI: 10.1016/j.jaad.2020.06.155

[8] Mahadevan U, Martin CF, Dubinsky M, Kane SV, Sands BE, Sandborn W. 960 exposure to anti-TNFα therapy in the third trimester of pregnancy is not associated with increased adverse outcomes: Results from the PIANO registry. Gastroenterology. 2014;**146**(5):S170. DOI: 10.1016/S0016-5085(14)60602-8

[9] Tan CS, Koralnik IJ. Progressive multifocal leukoencephalopathy and other disorders caused by JC virus: Clinical features and pathogenesis. The Lancet Neurology. 2010;**9**(4):425-437. DOI: 10.1016/S1474-4422(10)70040-5

[10] Van Der Heijde D, Deodhar A, FitzGerald O, et al. 4-year results from the RAPID-PsA phase 3 randomised placebo-controlled trial of certolizumab pegol in psoriatic arthritis. RMD Open. 2018;**4**(1). DOI: 10.1136/rmdopen-2017-000582

[11] Gottlieb AB, Blauvelt A, Thaçi D, et al. Certolizumab pegol for the treatment of chronic plaque psoriasis: Results through 48 weeks from 2 phase 3, multicenter, randomized, double-blinded, placebo-controlled studies (CIMPASI-1 and CIMPASI-2). Journal of the American Academy of Dermatology. 2018;**79**(2):302-314. DOI: 10.1016/j.jaad.2018.04.012

[12] Clowse ME, Förger F, Hwang C, et al. Minimal to no transfer of certolizumab pegol into breast milk: Results from CRADLE, a prospective, postmarketing, multicentre, pharmacokinetic study. Annals of the Rheumatic Diseases. 2017;**76**(11):1890-1896. DOI: 10.1136/annrheumdis-2017-211384

[13] Mariette X, Förger F, Abraham B, et al. Lack of placental transfer of certolizumab pegol during pregnancy: Results from CRIB, a prospective, postmarketing, pharmacokinetic study. Annals of the Rheumatic Diseases. 2018;**77**(2):228-233. DOI: 10.1136/annrheumdis-2017-212196

[14] Bagel J, Duffin KC, Moore A, et al. The effect of secukinumab on moderate-to-severe scalp psoriasis: Results of a 24-week, randomized, double-blind, placebo-controlled phase 3b study. Journal of the American Academy of Dermatology. 2017;**77**(4):667-674. DOI: 10.1016/j.jaad.2017.05.033

[15] Reich K, Sullivan J, Arenberger P, et al. Secukinumab shows high and sustained efficacy in nail psoriasis: 2.5-year results from the randomized placebo-controlled transfigure study. British Journal of Dermatology. 2020;**184**(3):425-436. DOI: 10.1111/bjd.19262

[16] Gottlieb AB, Kubanov A, Doorn MV, et al. Sustained efficacy of secukinumab in patients with moderate-to-severe palmoplantar psoriasis: 2·5-year results from GESTURE, a randomized, double-blind, placebo-controlled trial. British Journal of Dermatology. 2020;**182**(4):889-899. DOI: 10.1111/bjd.18331

[17] Bagel J, Nia J, Hashim PW, et al. Secukinumab is superior to ustekinumab in clearing skin in patients with moderate to severe plaque psoriasis (16-week CLARITY results). Dermatology and Therapy. 2018;**8**(4):571-579. DOI: 10.1007/s13555-018-0265-y

[18] Mease P, van der Heijde D, Landewé R, et al. Secukinumab improves active psoriatic arthritis symptoms and inhibits radiographic progression: Primary results from the randomised, double-blind, phase III FUTURE 5 study. Annals of the Rheumatic Diseases. 2018;**77**(6):890-897. DOI: 10.1136/annrheumdis-2017-212687

[19] Deodhar A, Mease PJ, McInnes IB, et al. Long-term safety of secukinumab in patients with moderate-to-severe plaque psoriasis, psoriatic arthritis, and ankylosing spondylitis: Integrated pooled clinical trial and post-marketing surveillance data. Arthritis Research & Therapy. 2019;**21**(1):111. DOI: 10.1186/s13075-019-1882-2

[20] Kimmel G, Chima M, Kim HJ, et al. Brodalumab in the treatment of moderate to severe psoriasis in patients when previous anti-interleukin 17A therapies have failed. Journal of the American Academy of Dermatology. 2019;**81**(3):857-859. DOI: 10.1016/j.jaad.2019.05.007

[21] Lebwohl M, Leonardi C, Wu JJ, et al. One-year pharmacovigilance update of brodalumab. Journal of Drugs in Dermatology. 2020;**19**(8):807-808. DOI: 10.36849/JDD.2020.5138

[22] Lebwohl MG, Papp KA, Marangell LB, et al. Psychiatric adverse events during treatment with brodalumab: Analysis of psoriasis clinical trials. Journal of the American Academy of Dermatology. 2018 Jan;**78**(1):81-89.e5. DOI: 10.1016/j.jaad.2017.08.024

[23] Paller AS, Seyger MMB, Magariños GA, et al. Efficacy and safety of ixekizumab in a phase III, randomized, double-blind, placebo-controlled study in paediatric patients with moderate-to-severe plaque psoriasis (IXORA-PEDS). British Journal of Dermatology. 2020;**183**(2):231-241. DOI: 10.1111/bjd.19147

[24] Blauvelt A, Leonardi C, Elewski B, et al. A head-to-head comparison of ixekizumab vs. guselkumab in patients with moderate-to-severe

plaque psoriasis: 24-week efficacy and safety results from a randomized, double-blinded trial. British Journal of Dermatology. 2021;**184**(6):1047-1058. DOI: 10.1111/bjd.19509

[25] Smolen JS, Sebba A, Ruderman E, et al. Op0228 efficacy and safety of ixekizumab versus adalimumab (spirit-H2h) with and without concomitant conventional synthetic disease-modifying antirheumatic drugs (dmard) in biologic dmard-naïve patients with psoriatic arthritis: 52-week results. Annals of the Rheumatic Diseases. 2020;**79**(Suppl 10):143-144. DOI: 10.1136/annrheumdis-2020-eular.4615

[26] Gordon KB, Blauvelt A, Papp KA, et al. Phase 3 trials of ixekizumab in moderate-to-severe plaque psoriasis. The New England Journal of Medicine. 2016;**375**(4):345-356. DOI: 10.1056/NEJMoa1512711

[27] Reich K, Warren RB, Lebwohl M, et al. Bimekizumab versus Secukinumab in Plaque Psoriasis. The New England Journal of Medicine. 2021;**385**(2):142-152. DOI: 10.1056/NEJMoa2102383

[28] Reich K, Papp KA, Blauvelt A, et al. Bimekizumab versus ustekinumab for the treatment of moderate to severe plaque psoriasis (BE VIVID): Efficacy and safety from a 52-week, multicentre, double-blind, active comparator and placebo controlled phase 3 trial. The Lancet. 2021;**397**(10273):487-498. DOI: 10.1016/S0140-6736(21)00125-2

[29] Blauvelt A, Papp KA, Griffiths CEM, et al. Efficacy and safety of guselkumab, an anti-interleukin-23 monoclonal antibody, compared with adalimumab for the continuous treatment of patients with moderate to severe psoriasis: Results from the phase III, double-blinded, placebo- and active comparator-controlled VOYAGE 1 trial. Journal of the American Academy of Dermatology. 2017;**76**(3):405-417. DOI: 10.1016/j.jaad.2016.11.041

[30] Reich K, Armstrong AW, Langley RG, et al. Guselkumab versus secukinumab for the treatment of moderate-to-severe psoriasis (ECLIPSE): Results from a phase 3, randomised controlled trial. The Lancet. 2019;**394**(10201):831-839. DOI: 10.1016/S0140-6736(19)31773-8

[31] Reich K, Armstrong AW, Foley P, et al. Efficacy and safety of guselkumab, an anti-interleukin-23 monoclonal antibody, compared with adalimumab for the treatment of patients with moderate to severe psoriasis with randomized withdrawal and retreatment: Results from the phase III, double-blind, placebo- and active comparator-controlled VOYAGE 2 trial. Journal of the American Academy of Dermatology. 2017;**76**(3):418-431. DOI: 10.1016/j.jaad.2016.11.042

[32] Papp K, Kimball A, Tyring S, et al. Maintenance of treatment response in chronic plaque psoriasis patients continuing treatment or discontinuing treatment with tildrakizumab in a 64-week, randomized controlled, phase 3 trial. Journal of the American Academy of Dermatology. 2017;**76**(6):AB164. DOI: 10.1016/j.jaad.2017.04.637

[33] Reich K, Warren RB, Iversen L, et al. Long-term efficacy and safety of tildrakizumab for moderate-to-severe psoriasis: Pooled analyses of two randomized phase III clinical trials (reSURFACE 1 and reSURFACE 2) through 148 weeks. British Journal of Dermatology. 2020;**182**(3):605-617. DOI: 10.1111/bjd.18232

[34] Reich K, Gooderham M, Thaçi D, et al. Risankizumab compared with adalimumab in patients with

moderate-to-severe plaque psoriasis (IMMvent): A randomised, double-blind, active-comparator-controlled phase 3 trial. Lancet. 2019;**394**(10198):576-586. DOI: 10.1016/S0140-6736(19)30952-3

[35] Gordon KB, Strober B, Lebwohl M, et al. Efficacy and safety of risankizumab in moderate-to-severe plaque psoriasis (UltIMMa-1 and UltIMMa-2): Results from two double-blind, randomised, placebo-controlled and ustekinumab-controlled phase 3 trials. Lancet. 2018;**392**(10148):650-661. DOI: 10.1016/S0140-6736(18)31713-6

[36] Warren RB, Blauvelt A, Poulin Y, et al. Efficacy and safety of risankizumab vs. secukinumab in patients with moderate-to-severe plaque psoriasis (IMMerge): Results from a phase III, randomized, open-label, efficacy–assessor-blinded clinical trial. British Journal of Dermatology. 2020;**184**(1):50-59. DOI: 10.1111/bjd.19341

[37] Gordon KB, Lebwohl M, Papp KA, et al. Long-term safety of risankizumab from 17 clinical trials in patients with moderate-to-severe plaque psoriasis. British Journal of Dermatology. 2022;**186**(3):466-475. DOI: 10.1111/bjd.20818

[38] Reich K, Rich P, Maari C, et al. Efficacy and safety of mirikizumab (LY3074828) in the treatment of moderate-to-severe plaque psoriasis: Results from a randomized phase II study. British Journal of Dermatology. 2019;**181**(1):88-95. DOI: 10.1111/bjd.17628

[39] Bissonnette R, Maari C, Menter M, et al. 15328 efficacy and safety of mirikizumab in patients with moderate to severe plaque psoriasis: 104-week results from a randomized phase 2 study. Journal of the American Academy of Dermatology. 2020;**83**(6):AB147. DOI: 10.1016/j.jaad.2020.06.677

[40] Kauffman CL, Aria N, Toichi E, et al. A phase I study evaluating the safety, pharmacokinetics, and clinical response of a human IL-12 p40 antibody in subjects with plaque psoriasis. The Journal of Investigative Dermatology. 2004;**123**(6):1037-1044. DOI: 10.1111/j.0022-202X.2004.23448.x

[41] Goel N, Stephens S. Certolizumab pegol. mAbs. 2010;**2**(2):137-147. DOI: 10.4161/mabs.2.2.11271

Chapter 6

Perspective Chapter: Role of Curcumin in the Management of Rheumatoid Arthritis and Psoriatic Arthritis

Km. Reena, Lalit Singh and Ritesh Kumar Tiwari

Abstract

Rheumatoid arthritis (RA) and psoriatic arthritis (PsA) are chronic inflammatory illnesses categorized by joint pain and swelling, along with systemic symptoms. The distinction between RA and PsA may be difficult to determine since their clinical presentations and symptoms are so similar. RA and PsA are treated in a palliative manner since they are not curable diseases. Allopathic medicines have serious side effects, and long term-consumption decreases patient quality of life. Hyperacidity, edema, stomach ulcers, gastrointestinal bleeding, perforation, and reduced appetite are some of the most common adverse effects. Curcumin, the primary active component within *Curcuma longa* (turmeric), has been demonstrated to be helpful in treating RA and PsA, with effectiveness attributed to its mode of activity. This chapter defines the correlation between RA and PsA and reports on the use and mechanism of curcumin in the management of these conditions. According to various literature surveys and evidence, it can be concluded that curcumin is a safe and effective therapeutic option for managing RA and PsA compared to synthetic medications.

Keywords: rheumatoid arthritis, psoriasis, psoriatic arthritis, curcumin, anti-inflammatory, Immunomodulator

1. Introduction

Rheumatoid arthritis (RA) is a severe immune-mediated condition that impacts more women than men and is most common among the elderly. In 2002, the prevalence rate was reported to range from 0.5–1% of the population, with geographical variation [1]. Synovial joint inflammation and deformity, and inflammation of surrounding tissues such as tendons, ligaments, and muscles, characterize this condition. Although RA is associated with an aberrant immune response, the basic causes and pathophysiology of the illness are still unknown. It is said to be induced by aberrant immune system responses as a consequence of numerous hereditary and environmental variables [2]. These immune system alterations might occur several years before patients begin to experience symptoms. RA damages the lining of synovial joints, causing increasing disability, early mortality, and economic hardship. Arthralgia, edema, and erythema, as well as reduction in degree of movement, are all symptoms of symmetrical joint activation [3]. Mild RA is defined as presence of symptoms for less than 6 months, while developed RA is defined as presence of symptoms for longer than 6 months. Joint inflammation and injury that worsens over time can lead to disability and a lower quality of life [4].

Psoriasis is an illness that mostly damages the skin or joints and affects 2–3% of the population. The heart, aorta, and lungs can also be impacted by the condition. The percentage among sufferers with psoriasis who progress to psoriatic arthritis (PsA) remains unclear, with rates varying from 6–42% in various studies. According to one comprehensive study, PsA impacts up to 24% of psoriasis sufferers. Psoriasis often develops 8 to 10 years before PsA. Because both RA and PsA are immune-mediated chronic inflammatory illnesses with similar pathophysiology, they should be treated together to reduce pharmaceutical adverse effects and costs [5].

PsA is a recurrent, inflammatory musculoskeletal condition that is associated with skin psoriasis and is seronegative. It affects men and women equally around the ages of 40 and 50 [6]. Peripheral and axial joints, enthesis, skin, and nails are among the organ system that are impacted. PsA is correlated with comorbidities including osteoporosis, uveitis, subclinical intestinal inflammation, and illness [7].

Identification of PsA has been challenging due to its heterogeneity. However, categorization parameters including CASPAR (ClASsification criteria for Psoriatic ARthritis) [8] as well as various screening methods have simplified the diagnostic process for general practitioners, dermatologists, and rheumatologists. Estimates of prevalence within the general population are quite variable, owing to variances in epidemiological study methods [9]. The estimated frequency of PsA ranges from 0.16 to 0.25% [10], according to updated categorization criteria. PsA is characterized by synovial hyperplasia, immune cell infiltration, and proliferation of both the skin and synovium. Ache, edema, and physical discomfort affect sufferers' ability to work effectively in everyday activities, leading to a decreased standard of living [11].

Both RA and PsA are severe inflammatory conditions marked by joint discomfort and edema as well as systemic symptoms. Both can cause joint injury as well as loss of function if not detected early. Consequently, early detection is critical for developing treatment methods that will improve therapeutic and radiological results [12].

Clinically, distinguishing between RA and PsA is complicated because their clinical presentations and symptoms are so similar. Both conditions are connected to prevalent varieties of arthritis, including gout or secondary osteoarthritis (OA), and share parallels with other inflammatory disorders [13].

Traditional medicine like curcumin has been used in conjunction with pharmaceuticals to manage RA and PsA. Treatment for these conditions aims to alleviate inflammation and prevent progression of the disease, including irreversible bone loss, preserve joint and muscle function, and reduce disease activation. Nonsteroidal anti-inflammatory drugs (NSAIDs), immunosuppressive agents, slow-acting antirheumatic drugs, immunological and biological agents, and botanicals are among the medications used.

First-line treatment to slow illness progression or decrease discomfort involves the use of biologic disease-modifying antirheumatic medications such as tocilizumab (an interleukin 6 (IL-6), sarilumab (an IL-6 inhibitor), or abatacept (an CD80/86 inhibitor). The mechanism of action of such medicines differs according to the drug used, but the main impact is to reduce inflammatory mediators and induce death in dysfunctional autoimmune cells. Despite their great efficacy, these drugs are hindered by their high costs [14]. NSAIDs are an alternative approach. Although these drugs are helpful exclusively for moderate instances of PsA, they cannot completely reduce symptoms [15].

Turmeric (*Curcuma longa*) is a curry spice as well as ancient Chinese therapeutic plant with anti-inflammatory applications. Components of turmeric include curcuminoids (curcumin, demethoxycurcumin, and bisdemethoxycurcumin), volatile oils (natlantone, tumerone, and zingiberone), proteins, carbohydrates, and resins. Turmeric regulates inflammation, cell development, and apoptosis, making it suitable for both prevention and treatment of various ailments due to its antioxidant and anti-inflammatory applications, along with its high safety profile, the bulk of which is attributed to curcumin [16]. Curcumin interacts with a wide variety of molecular domains, making it a pleiotropic chemical. According to in vitro and in vivo research, curcumin is a promising curative drug for various chronic illnesses, including pancreatitis, inflammatory bowel disease, chronic anterior uveitis, and certain malignancies. Curcumin's physiological actions or molecular processes have been explored in numerous cell and animal investigations, and research is ongoing. Curcumin has attracted attention as a possible RA treatment due to its antioxidant properties and regulatory role of associated inflammatory agents [17]. Curcumin is presently available as beverages, pills, capsules, lotions, gels, nasal sprays, extracts, and coloring additives for both food and medicinal applications. Even though several in vitro and in vivo investigations have demonstrated curcumin's safety and effectiveness profile, further placebo-controlled prospective studies are required before oral curcumin can be suggested as a viable therapy for RA and PsA.

2. Epidemiological characteristics of rheumatoid arthritis and psoriatic arthritis

RA and PsA have different epidemiological characteristics [18]. RA affects more than one million people in the United States [19], whereas PsA affects around half a million people [20]. Psoriasis affects roughly 30% of individuals [21]. RA and PsA are prevalent in different regions of the world. RA is common in various populations, with prevalence rates ranging from 0.5 and 1.0%; however, prevalence is significantly greater among Native American Indian communities (5–7%) but lower in China and Japan (0.2–7%) [22–24]. The ubiquity rate of PsA in the United States and Europe ranges from 0.1 to 0.4%, whereas it is lower in Japan. This diversity of incidence shows that risk of illness is impacted by both environmental and hereditary variables [25, 26].

3. Pathogenesis of rheumatoid arthritis and psoriatic arthritis

Clinically, RA and PsA are both comparable and distinct. This is probably due to underlying genetic variation, with some genes involved in pathogenesis being shared by both diseases and others contributing to each disease's unique pathogenesis [27]. According to studies, each illness is produced due to integrated and complicated signaling pathways that impact various immune responses that perform distinct roles in disease pathogenesis [28]. It is apparent that innate or adaptive immunological reactions are involved [29]. T cells, B cells, and the coordinated interplay of pro-inflammatory cytokines all play important roles in the pathogenesis of RA. In PsA, activated T lymphocytes and macrophages perform a crucial function [30].

3.1 Rheumatoid arthritis

RA susceptibility is mostly determined by genetic factors, with heritability varying between 50 and 60%. More than 30% of genetic risk is accounted for by the human leukocyte antigen (HLA) locus, while non-HLA genes, such as tumor necrosis factor-alpha (TNF-alpha), have also been identified [31]. The pathophysiology of RA is characterized by a complex interaction between the adaptive and innate immune systems, as well as inflammatory infiltrates in the synovium and synovial fluid. Key contributors to the disease include dendritic cells, mast cells, neutrophils, and macrophages. T cells and B cells generate cytokines, antibodies, and immunological complexes, with the onset of RA attributed to phosphoinositide-3-kinase (PI3K) delta and gamma signaling molecules associated with T cells and B cells, as well as neutrophil and mast cell activity. The production of pro-inflammatory cytokines and chemokines, along with dysregulation of three essential T-helper (TH) cell subtypes—TH1, TH17, and regulatory T (Treg) cells—play crucial roles in the initiation and progression of RA [32].

3.2 Psoriatic arthritis

According to family research, the genes linked with PsA are HLA-CW*0602, IL-23r, and IL-12b [33]. The unavailability of established genetic vulnerability sites may also be associated with reduced incidence and greater variability of PsA [34]. Genetically predisposed people who have a dysfunctional immune response are hypothesized to develop PsA, resulting in immune cell infiltration and cytokine production. Infiltrating cells such as activated T cells and macrophages are assumed to perform a key role in generating inflammatory or inflammatory and degenerative events within joint tissues, along with skin psoriasis [35]. Inflammatory cytokines released via T cells, including IL-1, IL-2, IL-10, interferon (IFN), and tumor necrosis factor (TNF), are abundant in the synovium [36]. Development of PsA is linked to the IL-22 and IL-23/Th17 axis [37]. In matched PsA synovial tissue and skin samples, the expression of IL-17 genes was higher in the skin compared to the synovium, but the overexpression of TNF pathway was equivalent between both sites. The expression of angiogenesis-related genes and IL-6 was elevated in the synovium but not in the skin [38]. According to an assessment of PsA etiology, there may be four clinical phenotypes that are determined by genotype: synovial predominant, entheseal predominant, axial predominant, and mutilans [39].

4. Difference between rheumatoid arthritis and psoriatic arthritis

RA is characterized as an immune-mediated, persistent, inflammatory condition that causes symptoms like synovitis, cartilage degeneration, and bone destruction. PsA is also an autoimmune systemic illness characterized by numerous radiological symptoms [40]. **Table 1** lists the features of RA and PsA.

5. Clinical characteristics of rheumatoid arthritis and psoriatic arthritis

RA categorization guidelines were created by the American College of Rheumatology (ACR) and the European League Against Rheumatism (ELAR) for patient identification or application in the clinical trials [42]. Confirmation of unambiguous, persistent clinical synovitis in at least one joint is the most important

Features	Rheumatoid arthritis	Psoriatic arthritis
No. of affected joints	30–50% with arthritis	Predominant: polyarthritis
Contribution of joints	like distal interphalangeal joints is the examle.	Usually, distal interphalangeal joints
Enthesitis	Typically, medically diagnosed in 60–80%	Not typical
Dactylitis	Present in 30%	Not typical
Axial involvement	Axial spondylarthritis phenotypes	Erosive cervical disease
Skin, nail disease	80% in psoriasis and 60% in nail disease	Reduced community threat or background threat
Serology	RF and CCP are generally negative	RF or CCP are generally positive
Radiographic alterations	Periosteal new bone formation (uncommon especially in early disease)	Erosion or osteopenia

CCP = cyclic citrullinated peptide, RF = rheumatoid factor.
Adapted from: [41].

Table 1.
Differentiating rheumatoid arthritis from psoriatic arthritis.

clinical feature of RA. The number of afflicted joints, duration of symptoms, and existence of serological indicators or an increased acute-phase reactant round out the criteria for RA. PsA classification criteria are used to classify individuals having inflammatory articular illness for clinical studies in psoriatic arthritis [43]. Psoriasis, psoriatic arthritis, psoriatic nail degradation, and dactylitis are all important clinical features. Neither categorization nor diagnostic criteria should be conflated. In RA, joint involvement is generally symmetric, but joint association in PsA is frequently. Individuals with RA mostly experience polyarthritis (five joints affected), however joint involvement can also be oligoarticular or polyarticular [44].

RA usually affects the wrists, shoulders, elbows, and metacarpophalangeal joints. PsA usually affects the distal interphalangeal joints of the hands and feet, major joints of lower extremities, the axial spine, and sacroiliac joints, as well as the metacarpophalangeal joints. Due to the potential damage to the axial skeleton by PsA, it is classified within the spondylarthritis spectrum rather than as RA. This includes involvement of areas such as the sacroiliac joint and spine [45].

About 35% of individuals with PsA experience enthesis (inflammation of attachment points of tendons or ligaments), but enthesis is rare in RA [46]. In PsA, dactylitis (inflammation of whole digit) is a frequent symptom, occurring in approximately 50% of sufferers. Dactylitis affects only around 5% of RA sufferers [47].

Extra-articular symptoms of RA and PsA include ocular problems [48]. Keratoconjunctivitis sicca is a frequent ocular symptom of RA, affecting about 18% of individuals [49].

Both RA and PsA cause cutaneous symptoms. Rheumatoid nodules, vasculitis skin lesions, and granulomatous dermatoses are the most frequent cutaneous manifestations of RA. In 84% of patient with PsA, skin symptoms manifest before or predate the appearance of joint problems. Approximately 96% of people with PsA either present with or have a history of and even a genetic background of psoriasis [50, 51].

6. Diagnosis of rheumatoid arthritis and psoriatic arthritis

6.1 Rheumatoid arthritis

Two indicators commonly used for diagnosing RA are anti-cyclic citrullinated antibodies (anti-CCP) and rheumatoid factor (RF). Meta-analysis studies suggest that anti-CCP exhibits either identical or greater sensitivity (67% for anti-CCP vs. 69% for RF) and greater specificity (95% for anti-CCP vs. 85% for RF) compared to RF. Moreover, anti-CCP has a stronger predictive value for the onset of erosive illness. It is important to note that while RF and anti-CCP are highly specific, they can also be found in a wide range of other illnesses [52].

In patients with RA, antinuclear antibodies (ANAs) and anti-double-stranded DNA (anti-dsDNA) antibodies are commonly detected. However, it is worth considering that the use of TNF monoclonal antibodies like infliximab for managing RA may elevate the serum concentration of ANA and anti-dsDNA [53].

6.2 Psoriatic arthritis

Diagnosing PsA can be challenging because of the many similarities between it and other rheumatological diseases such as RA, OA, and gout. Furthermore, between 10 and 15% of undiagnosed psoriatic patients in dermatological clinics are undiagnosed, with a delay in diagnosis also connected with poorer disease outcomes [54]. In theory, diagnostic testing for PsA is not available; instead, individuals are diagnosed depending only clinical features. Symptoms are typically diverse, with "domains" such as peripheral arthritis, enthesitis, dactylitis, axial illness, psoriasis, and nail diseases occurring frequently [55].

7. Comorbidities associated with rheumatoid arthritis and psoriatic arthritis

Comorbidities associated with autoimmune inflammatory illnesses include infections, cancer, depression and anxiety, cardiovascular difficulties, non-alcohol fatty liver disease (NAFLD), and obesity [56].

Table 2 lists important comorbidities associated with RA and PsA.

S.no	Comorbidities	Rheumatoid arthritis	Psoriatic arthritis
1.	Cardiovascular	RA is associated with an increased risk of cardiovascular illness, with the greatest incidence occurring among the elderly [57]. There has been evidence of a heightened incidence of atrial fibrillation, stroke, and hypertension [58]. Even after accounting for frequent cardiovascular comorbidities or risk factors, systemic inflammation increases the potential of cardiovascular mortality in RA sufferers [59].	PsA is associated with a greater incidence of myocardial infraction, angina, and hypertension [60]. Level of severity of PsA is a major determinant of cardiovascular morbidity, along with established risk factors for cardiovascular conditions such as diabetes and hyperlipidemia.

S.no	Comorbidities	Rheumatoid arthritis	Psoriatic arthritis
2.	Malignancies	Increase in non-Hodgkin's lymphoma, Hodgkin's condition, cancer of lungs and skin cancer of nonmelanoma, were reported in a investigation of 20,699 individuals with rheumatoid arthritis between 1977 and 1987, previous studies demonstrate link among rheumatoid arthritis and non-Hodgkin's lymphoma, Hodgkin's disease, lung cancer [61]. Other community-based studies found that smoking-related malignancies are 20–50% more likely and nonmelanoma skin cancer is 470% more likely in patients with RA. The majority of cancers are linked to psoriasis and RA not PsA, indicating a disease-specific relationship. Several variables, including patient characteristics [62], illness features, and lifestyle factors, all have an impact [63].	In a cohort study of PsA, around 10.2% of participants got cancer; however, this rate does not vary from the rate of cancer in the overall community [64]. Malignant neoplasms were shown to be the third leading cause of mortality (17.0%) in patients with PsA [65], after cardiovascular and respiratory system illnesses [65].
3.	Nonalcoholic fatty liver disease (NAFLD)	NAFLD affects 10–24% of people in the normal community whereas it impacts 57.5–74% of the obese population [66]. According to the analysis of autopsy histologic liver discomfort in RA patients, fatty alterations were seen in 42 of 182 cases (23%) [67].	PsA was demonstrated to be a determinant of NAFLD in individuals with psoriasis in an Italian study [68] regardless of age, gender, BMI, or obesity.

Table 2.
Comorbidities associated with rheumatoid arthritis and psoriatic arthritis.

8. Treatment of rheumatoid arthritis and psoriatic arthritis

Treatment methods for RA and PsA may differ due to variations in disease etiology and therapeutic response. Medications that target upstream factors like TNF seem to be beneficial for both PsA and RA. However, medications targeting downstream cytokines show high condition-specific efficacy. For example, targeting IL-6 is highly effective in RA, while targeting IL-17A is effective in PsA but not necessarily in both diseases.

Disease-modifying antirheumatic drugs (DMARDS) have long been utilized for managing rheumatological diseases, but their long-term therapeutic benefits in PsA are primarily based on clinical experience rather than comprehensive trial-based study. PsA can be treated with a number of approaches, including nonpharmacological approaches such as weight loss, smoking cessation, and exercise. NSAIDs and corticosteroid injections are utilized to alleviate symptoms.

8.1 Nonsteroidal anti-inflammatory drugs

Patients benefit from treatment with NSAIDS for alleviation of symptoms, but NSAIDs do not completely resolve or stop joint deterioration or the psoriatic component of PsA [69]. Indeed, no changes in psoriasis area severity index (PASI) score or erythrocyte sedimentation rate (ESR) were identified in controlled investigations [70].

8.2 Conventional synthetic disease-modifying antirheumatic drugs

For the management of RA, methotrexate is the most prescribed conventional synthetic disease-modifying antirheumatic medication (csDMARD). Methotrexate is reported to decrease disease intensity and increase quality of life in individuals with PsA. Leflunomide has proven to be more effective than placebo in treating patients with PsA [71].

8.3 Biologic disease-modifying antirheumatic drugs

8.3.1 TNF-α inhibitors

TNF-α is a proinflammatory cytokine overexpressed in the synovium of inflammatory arthritis patients. The US Food and Drug Administration (FDA) has approved five TNF inhibitors for the treatment of RA and PsA: etanercept, infliximab, adalimumab, golimumab, and certolizumab pegol. TNF inhibition in RA inhibits bone degradation as well as reduces injury via reducing osteoclast production to decrease systemic inflammation. TNF-α inhibitor's capacity to prevent the production of matrix metalloproteinases and aggrecanases has been proposed as a way to decrease cartilage matrix degradation. TNF-α inhibitors diminish synoviocyte hyperproliferation and T-cell and microphage infiltration in PsA, decreasing synovial thickness. TNF-α inhibitors control angiogenesis and osteoclastogenesis in PsA and decrease synovitis [72].

Inhibitors of IL-17A target various immune cells including T helper (Th) 17 cells, macrophages, mast cells, dendritic cells, natural killer cells, and CD8+ T cells, all of which release IL-17A, a proinflammatory effector cytokine. PsA patients had increased levels of IL-17A in their synovial fluid, which has been linked to pathogenic angiogenesis, osteoclastogenesis, and fibrogenesis in studies. Interactions between IL-17A and synovial-like fibroblast, osteoblast, and osteoclast precursors encouraged persistent inflammation and bone alterations in PsA, which contribute to joint destruction 91. Osteoclastogenesis, upregulated matrix metalloproteinases, and another proinflammatory cytokines can also be induced by TNF-α and IL-17. The existence of IL-17-generating T cells in PsA patients is linked to illness performance markers (such as CRP and ESR) or radiographic degradation. Secukinumab and oxekizumab, both IL-17A inhibitors, have been approved by the FDA for the management of active PsA [73].

8.3.1.1 IL-12 and IL-23 dual inhibitor

IL-12 and IL-23 are two key cytokines associated with the progression of psoriasis and PsA. In response to inflammation, monocytes or macrophages release IL-12, which stimulates Th1 cells, while myeloid dendritic cells produce IL-23, a cytokine that regulates the activity of Th17 cells [74]. IL-12 aids in the differentiation of Th1 cells and the activation of natural killer (NK) cells, while IL-23 is linked to osteoclastogenesis and bone degradation.

Ustekinumab, an inhibitor of the IL-12/23p40 subunit, blocks Th1 and Th17 differentiation and downstream IL-17 production. Phase III clinical studies have shown that ustekinumab significantly reduces the radiographic progression of joint damage and improves clinical symptoms in individuals with active PsA [75].

However, ustekinumab has not been found to be effective in individuals with RA. Similarly, guselkumab, a specific inhibitor of IL-23, has shown ineffectiveness in individuals with RA, although initial results in patients with PsA suggest it may help with joint pain. Further research is needed.

In a phase II study of PsA, risankizumab, a specific inhibitor of IL-23, has shown promising effects [76].

8.3.1.2 IL-6 inhibitors

In acute-phase inflammatory reactions, macrophages and T cells generate IL-6, a proinflammatory cytokine. IL-6, like transforming growth factor and IL-23, helps to keep pathogenic Th17 cells differentiated and produce IL-17. IL-6 levels in the synovium have been found to be elevated in individuals with active RA and PsA [77]. Tocilizumab or sarilumab, two IL-6 inhibitors approved by the FDA for the management of RA, decrease illness activity and radiographic joint damage. For the treatment of RA, further IL-6 inhibitors (such as olokizumab) are being developed [78].

8.3.1.3 T-cell activation inhibitors

Abatacept, a fusion protein that interacts with CD80/CD86 ligands on the surfaces of antigen-presenting cells, works by suppressing T-cell stimulation and reducing levels of proinflammatory cytokines and autoantibodies. The FDA has approved abatacept for the management of active RA, particularly in individuals who have not responded well to TNF inhibitors. Additionally, the FDA has authorized abatacept for the management of active PsA. Findings from a phase III trial have demonstrated the effectiveness of abatacept, regardless of prior exposure to TNF inhibitors. However, it is worth noting that in individuals with both psoriasis and PsA, abatacept did not improve skin symptoms compared to placebo [79].

8.3.1.4 CD20 inhibitors

B cells play a significant role in RA by generating autoantibodies, which are immune proteins that mistakenly target and react with a person's own tissues or organs. Additionally, B cells produce various cytokines and express the receptor activator of nuclear factor kappa B ligand (RANKL), which promotes the development and activation of osteoclasts. B cells express CD20 molecules, and inhibiting them leads to B cell loss and direct downregulation of RANKL and proinflammatory cytokines.

Rituximab, a CD20 inhibitor, is approved by the FDA for the treatment of RA in individuals who have not responded to TNF inhibitors when used in conjunction with methotrexate. Clinical trials have shown the efficacy of rituximab in treating RA. However, rituximab has not been found to be helpful in individuals with PsA, possibly because they lack circulating autoantibodies [80].

8.4 Targeted synthetic oral small-molecule disease-modifying drugs

8.4.1 Phosphodiesterase-4-inhibitors

Phosphodiesterase-4 (PDE4) is an enzyme that increases cyclic adenosine monophosphate breakdown, upregulating inflammatory responses by increasing levels of cytokines such as TNF-α, IL-12, and IL-23. Apremilast, a PDE4 inhibitor, is approved by the FDA for the management of active PsA. Approval was based on data from phase III human trials that showed apremilast reduced disease activity and improved clinical outcomes. There have been no studies evaluating apremilast's potential to slow radiographic progression. Apremilast was demonstrated to decrease TNF release from human rheumatoid synovial membrane cells and diminish clinical disease activity in animal models of RA. Furthermore, in a phase II trial of individuals with RA, apremilast was shown to be ineffective when compared to placebo [81].

8.4.1.1 Janus kinase inhibitors

Janus kinases (JAKs) are cytoplasmic tyrosine kinases that control inflammatory cytokine signaling, such as IL-2, IL-4, IL-7, IL-9, IL-15, and IL-21, therefore regulating immune responses. Tofacitinib is approved by the FDA for the management of individuals with active RA who have an inadequate response to or cannot tolerate methotrexate. Treatment with tofacitinib was linked to a reduction in active disease signs and symptoms, enhancement of physical as well as wellbeing condition of life, and a reduction in radiographic progress among individuals with RA in clinical trials. Tofacitinib was found to be effective for both PsA and psoriasis in the phase III Oral Psoriatic Arthritis Trial (OPAL). Tofacitinib's safety profile was similar among individuals with RA and individuals with PsA. The FDA approved tofacitinib for the treatment of PsA in 2017 [81].

9. Curcumin importance for management of rheumatoid arthritis and psoriatic arthritis

Curcumin, an antioxidant, anti-inflammatory, and immune-modulatory agent, is found in turmeric. It has been found to assist with arthritis and joint pain. Given that persistent inflammation is a key feature of arthritis, it is important to note that curcumin has been reported to be beneficial for both inflammatory bowel disease (IBD) and irritable bowel syndrome (IBS). Additionally, curcumin may potentially help reduce neuroinflammation associated with Alzheimer's disease. Recent studies suggest that curcuminoids, when combined with black pepper, may help alleviate the painful joint symptoms associated with RA, PsA, or OA.

PsA is a type of inflammatory arthritis that is similar to RA but with significant differences. PsA results in shiny, red spots on the skin, often known as "plaques." Psoriatic symptoms are frequently asymmetric, which means that if one wrist hurts, the other may be symptom free. Curcumin can help the immune response by reducing inflammation, which can help to alleviate joint discomfort, increase mobility, and restore functioning in troublesome regions. Curcumin's anti-inflammatory properties have been proven in several trials, including investigations of back pain, muscular discomfort, and inflammation associated with asthma and allergies.

The antiarthritic effect of curcumin has been investigated in patients with RA. In one study, 45 participants was randomly allocated to one of three groups: treatment with 500 mg of curcumin, treatment with 50 mg of diclofenac sodium, or a combination of the two. The Disease Activity Scores (DAS) of patients across all three groups showed significant statistical improvement. However, the curcumin group showed superior results and had the highest percentage of recovery. According to the American College of Rheumatology (ACR) score, the curcumin group also exhibited the greatest reduction in pain and joint edema. Curcumin has been demonstrated to be safe and effective in treating RA [80]. **Figure 1** shows the effect of curcumin on RA and PsA.

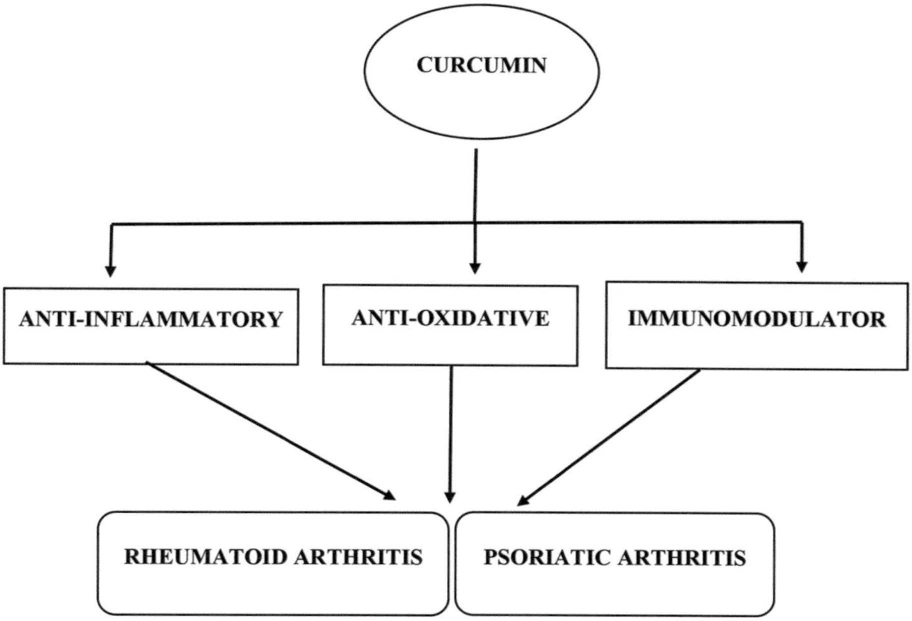

Figure 1.
Effect of curcumin on rheumatoid and psoriatic arthritis.

10. Mechanism of curcumin in the management of rheumatoid arthritis and psoriatic arthritis

Curcumin has great potential for managing both RA and PsA via different mechanisms.

10.1 Rheumatoid arthritis

Arthritis produces inflammation and discomfort, yet its root cause is unknown; thus, treatment of its underlying causes is challenging. Current therapies for arthritis focus on alleviating joint pain resulting from inflammation, normal wear and tear, and muscle pain. Steroids, painkillers, and NSAIDs are commonly prescribed to manage arthritis symptoms, reducing inflammation and extreme pain. However, their long-term use is discouraged due to inadequate pain relief, immunological abnormalities, and significant gastrointestinal and cardiovascular side effects. Therefore, there is a need for herbal treatments with anti-inflammatory properties, especially in managing conditions like RA and OA, given the withdrawal of several FDA-approved anti-inflammatory medications. Phytomedicines and chemical compounds derived from plants have attracted global interest for their potential in managing various debilitating diseases [81].

In addition to its use as a cooking spice, curcumin may be utilized as an alternative treatment for arthritis. It has traditionally been used in Chinese and Ayurvedic medicine as an anti-inflammatory therapy.

Curcumin has shown positive immunomodulatory effects by reducing the generation of pro-inflammatory cytokines as well as dysregulated immune cell activities in RA, including TH1, TH17, and regulatory T (Treg), and B cells. Curcumin has been found to reduce the severity of RA complications by inhibiting the production of pro-inflammatory mediators such as nuclear factor-B (NF-B), activator protein-1 (AP-1), and mitogen-activated protein kinases (MAPKs) in immune cells and synovial fibroblast cells. Curcumin also affects the expression of energy-related transcription factors, including signal transducer and activator of transcription, peroxisome proliferator-activated receptor-c, activator protein-1, cAMP responding element binding protein, estrogen response element, and others. Consequently, turmeric as well its constituents are claimed to possess anti-inflammatory, anti-diabetic, and anti-lipidemic properties. In several types of cultured cells and animal experiments, extracts from the roots of *Curcuma longa* have demonstrated potential anti-inflammatory, antioxidant, chemopreventive, and chemotherapeutic action. Curcumin has also been found to help with a variety of clinical problems, including cancer, inflammatory illness, and digestive issues. However, according to several studies, taking curcumin orally lowers its bioavailability considerably. The iontophoretic technique, which is based on the electromagnetic principle and employs direct electrical current, has been utilized in physiotherapy to improve intradermal medication delivery [82].

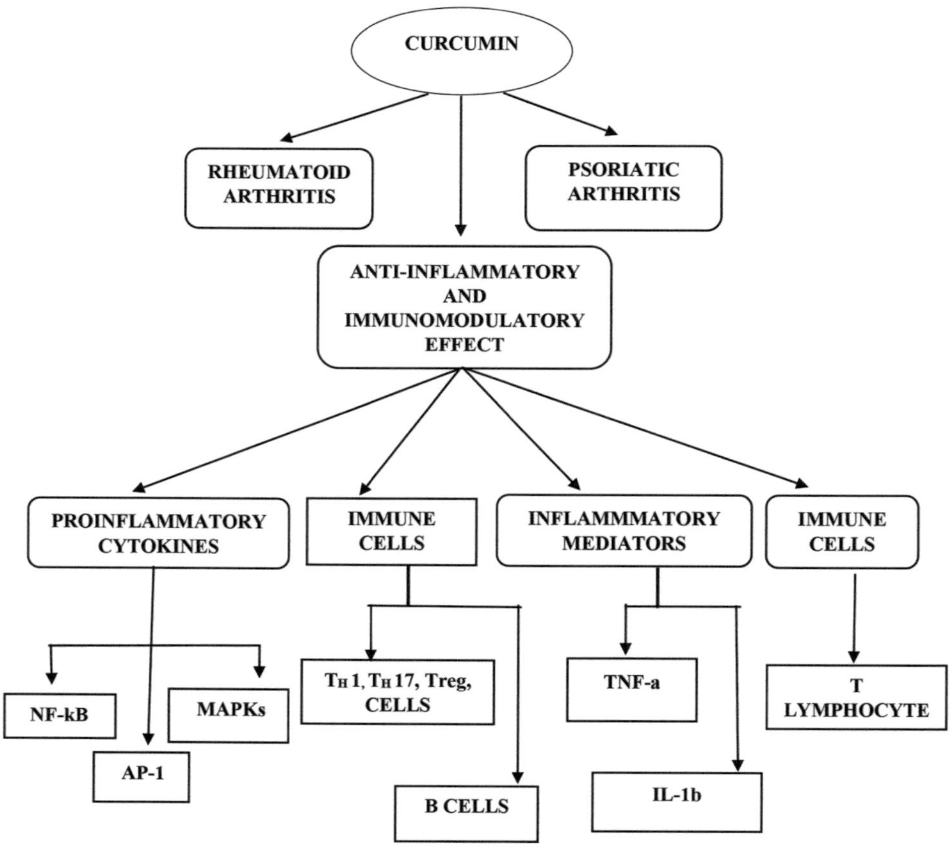

Figure 2.
Diagrammatic representation for mechanism of curcumin in rheumatoid and psoriatic arthritis.

10.2 Psoriatic arthritis

Curcumin inhibits the action of nuclear factor kappa B (NF-kB) and various inflammatory markers, including tumor necrosis factor-alpha (TNF-a) and interleukin-6 (IL-6). Additionally, it can alleviate discomfort associated with immune-mediated inflammatory diseases, aside from its anti-inflammatory properties.

Studies have demonstrated that curcumin reduces inflammation and symptoms associated with autoimmune collagen-induced arthritis (CIA), which is a common animal model used to study RA. These beneficial effects of curcumin may be attributed to its immunomodulatory action via modulation of T lymphocytes.

Combining acupuncture in the style of Chinese medicine with a daily intake of 500 mg turmeric (*Curcuma longa* root extract) along with 3 mg of black pepper extract (*Piper nigrum*), standardized to contain 95% curcuminoid and 425 mg of sarsaparilla root (*Smilax officinalis*) in powdered capsules may potentially alleviate symptoms of PsA and maintain them at a manageable level. PsA can be addressed with a treatment regimen that includes acupuncture, turmeric, sarsaparilla root, and vitamin D3. **Figure 2** depicts the mechanism through which curcumin acts on both RA and PsA.

11. Various in vivo and in vitro studies have demonstrated the role of curcumin in the management of rheumatoid and psoriatic arthritis

Table 3 lists some of the studies demonstrating the role of curcumin in managing RA and PsA.

S.R.NO	Researcher	Work done	References
1.	Amin et al.	Study of curcumin's impact on experimentally generated arthritis of the temporomandibular joint. Results show curcumin may be useful as an antioxidant agent for inflammatory and degenerative conditions like arthritis.	[81]
2.	Skyvalidas et al.	Study investigating curcumin's ability to decrease the production of IFN and IL-17 in psoriasis and PsA patients' peripheral blood mononuclear cells. Results show that curcumin reduces pro-inflammatory IFN and IL-17 production in vitro in psoriatic illness, suggesting its potential as a dietary immunosuppressant in such individuals.	[82]
3.	Martin et al.	Study of natural medicine therapy in a patient with PsA. Acupuncture, turmeric (*C. longa*), sarsaparilla (*S. officinalis*), and vitamin D may all be effective natural treatments for PsA, as these methods were able to alleviate the patient's PsA symptoms and keep them at a manageable level.	[83]
4.	Manca et al.	Study of curcumin-loaded hyalurosomes for RA. The ability of these vesicles to downregulate the production of anti-apoptotic proteins IAP1 and IAP2 and stimulate the production of IL-10 while reducing the production of IL-6 and IL-15 and reactive oxygen species was demonstrated in vitro using fibroblast-like synovial cells cultured in synovial fluid. The results suggest the potential use of curcumin-loaded hyalurosomes in controlling the local consequences of RA.	[84]

S.R.NO	Researcher	Work done	References
5.	Wang et al.	Study of curcumin's therapeutic benefits and pharmacological mechanism in collagen-induced arthritis (CIA) rats. Results show that curcumin has a substantial pharmacological action in lowering the inflammatory response in macrophages and has therapeutic benefits in CIA rats. Its mechanism might be linked to the inhibition of the NF-B signaling pathway and induction of macrophage apoptosis.	[85]
6.	Dewangan et al.	Study of the effectiveness of curcumin-loaded carboxymethyl cellulose acetate butyrate (CMCAB) polymer and the development of well-defined nanoparticles, which improve CUR-CMCAB nanoparticle solubility for RA therapy. It may also be inferred that several phytochemicals, including curcumin, can deliver effective treatments without the negative effects associated with routinely used drugs if properly produced as pharmaceuticals employing specialized carrier systems.	[86]
7.	Jeengar et al.	Study of the capacity of emu oil to penetrate the skin and boost the antiarthritic potential of lipophilic bioactive curcumin, which has weak permeability across biological membranes. In arthritic animals, topical treatment of a curcumin–emu oil combination resulted in significantly lower levels of pro-inflammatory mediators TNF-, IL-1, and IL-6 ($p = 0.05$, 0.001, and 0.01 1). Topical administration of curcumin with emu oil has the potential to be a noninvasive and effective therapy for inflammatory arthritis.	[87]

Table 3.
Various in vivo and in vitro studies demonstrating the role of curcumin in the management of rheumatoid and psoriatic arthritis.

12. Conclusion

RA and PsA are both chronic inflammatory, autoimmune conditions that are treated in a palliative manner because they are incurable. The production and use of drugs derived from chemical compounds can have serious negative effects, with long-term usage often decreasing overall quality of life. Curcumin, a compound found in natural vegetation, has garnered attention worldwide for its potential in managing various debilitating diseases. Specifically, it has shown effectiveness in treating RA and PsA. Curcumin interacts with receptors associated with the pathophysiology of these diseases, helping to alleviate symptoms. Arthritis, characterized by persistent inflammation in multiple joints, can be difficult to diagnose due to its chronic nature. Accurate diagnosis is crucial because differences in underlying pathophysiology and medication tolerance can significantly impact treatment outcomes. Curcumin has proven beneficial in effectively treating both diseases without adverse side effects, potentially leading to symptom improvement in both conditions.

Acknowledgements

I acknowledge Invertis University, Bareilly, Pharmacy, for providing the necessary requirement for the accomplishment of this work, I am extremely grateful to our chairmen DR. Umesh Gautam sir for giving me the golden oppurtinity for completion of this article.

Conflict of interest

The author has no conflict of interest, financial or otherwise.

Consent for publication

Not applicable.

Author details

Km. Reena[1*], Lalit Singh[2] and Ritesh Kumar Tiwari[3]

1 Department of Pharmacy, Invertis University, Bareilly, UP, India

2 Faculty of Pharmacy, Future Institute of Medical Sciences, UP, India

3 Department of Pharmacy, Shriram Murti Smarak College of Engineering and Technology, UP, India

*Address all correspondence to: yadavreena2807@gmail.com

References

[1] Silman AJ, Pearson JE. Epidemiology and genetics of rheumatoid arthritis. Arthritis Research. 2002;**4**(2):265-272

[2] Symmons D, Turner G, Webb R, Asten P, Barrett E, Lunt M, et al. The prevalence of rheumatoid arthritis in the United Kingdom: New estimates for a new century. Rheumatology. 2002;**41**(7):793-800

[3] van der Linden MP et al. Long-term impact of delay in assessment of patients with early arthritis. Arthritis and Rheumatism. 2010;**62**(12):3537-3546

[4] Cai Q, Xin Z, Zuo L, Li F, Liu B. Alzheimer's disease and rheumatoid arthritis: A Mendelian randomization study. Frontiers in Neuroscience. 2018;**12**:627

[5] Feletar M, Foley P, Brown MA. Developments in psoriasis and psoriatic arthritis. Drug Discovery Today: Disease Mechanisms. 2008;**5**:47-54

[6] Chimenti MS, Ballanti E, Perricone C, Cipriani P, Giacomelli R, Perricone R. Immunomodulation in psoriatic arthritis: Focus on cellular and molecular pathways. Autoimmunity. 2013;**12**(5):599-606

[7] Sukhov A, Adamopoulos IE, Maverakis E. Interactions of the immune system with skin and bone tissue in psoriatic arthritis: A comprehensive review. Clinical Reviews in Allergy and Immunology. 2016;**51**(1):87-99

[8] Taylor W, Gladman D, Helliwell P, et al. Classification criteria for psoriatic arthritis: Development of new criteria from a large international study. Arthritis and Rheumatism. 2006;**54**(8):2665-2673

[9] Alamanos Y, Voulgari PV, Drosos AA. Incidence and prevalence of psoriatic arthritis: A systematic review. The Journal of Rheumatology. 2008;**35**(7):1354-1358

[10] Gelfand JM, Gladman DD, Mease PJ, Smith N, Margolis DJ, Nijsten T, et al. Epidemiology of psoriatic arthritis in the population of the United States. Journal of the American Academy of Dermatology. 2005;**53**(4):573

[11] Prey S, Paul C, Bronsard V, Puzenat E, Gourraud PA, Aractingi S, et al. Assessment of risk of psoriatic arthritis in patients with plaque psoriasis: A systematic review of the literature. Journal of the European Academy of Dermatology and Venereology. 2010;**24**(2):31-35

[12] Villeneuve E, Nam JL, Bell MJ, et al. A systematic literature review of strategies promoting early referral and reducing delays in the diagnosis and management of inflammatory arthritis. Annals of the Rheumatic Diseases. 2013;**72**(1):12-22

[13] Gladman DD. Clinical features and diagnostic considerations in psoriatic arthritis. Rheumatic Disease Clinics of North America. 2015;**41**(4):569-579

[14] Joshi P, Dhaneshwar SS. An update on disease modifying antirheumatic drugs. Inflammation & Allergy Drug Targets. 2014;**13**(4):249-261

[15] Mease PJ, Armstrong AW. Managing patients with psoriatic disease: The diagnosis and pharmacologic treatment of psoriatic arthritis in patients with psoriasis. Drugs. 2014;**74**(4):423-441

[16] Gupta SC, Patchva S, Koh W, Aggarwal BB. Discovery of curcumin,

a component of golden spice, and its miraculous biological activities. Clinical and Experimental Pharmacology & Physiology. 2012;**39**(3):283-299

[17] Kloesch B, Becker T, Dietersdorfer E, Kiener H, Steiner G. Anti-inflammatory and apoptotic effects of the polyphenol curcumin on human fibroblast-like synoviocytes. International Immunopharmacology. 2013;**15**(2):400-405

[18] Koeberle A, Werz O. Multi-target approach for natural products in inflammation. Drug Discovery Today. 2014;**19**(12):1871-1882

[19] Behrens F, Koehm M, Thaçi D, et al. Anti-citrullinated protein antibodies are linked to erosive disease in an observational study of patients with psoriatic arthritis. Rheumatology. 2016;**55**(10):1791-1795

[20] Helmick CG, Felson DT, Lawrence RC, et al. Estimates of the prevalence of arthritis and other rheumatic conditions in the United States: Part I. Arthritis & Rheumatism. 2008;**58**(1):15-25

[21] Gelfand JM, Gladman DD, Mease PJ, et al. Epidemiology of psoriatic arthritis in the population of the United States. Journal of the American Academy of Dermatology. 2005;**53**(4):553-573

[22] Mease PJ, Gladman DD, Papp KA, et al. Prevalence of rheumatologist-diagnosed psoriatic arthritis in patients with psoriasis in European/North American dermatology clinics. Journal of the American Academy of Dermatology. 2013;**69**(5):729-735

[23] Shichikawa K, Inoue K, Hirota S, et al. Changes in the incidence and prevalence of rheumatoid arthritis in Kamitonda, Wakayama, Japan, 1965-1996. Annals of the Rheumatic Diseases. 1999;**58**(12):751-756

[24] Zeng Q, Huang S, Chen R. 10-year epidemiological study on rheumatic diseases in Shantou area. Zhonghua Nei Ke Za Zhi. 1997;**36**(3):193-197

[25] Hunter TM, Boytsov NN, Zhang X, et al. Prevalence of rheumatoid arthritis in the United States adult population in healthcare claims databases, 2004-2014. Rheumatology International. 2017;**37**(9):1551-1557

[26] Alamanos Y, Voulgari PV, Drosos AA. Incidence and prevalence of psoriatic arthritis: A systematic review. The Journal of Rheumatology. 2008;**35**(7):1354-1358

[27] Nograles KE, Davidovici B, Krueger JG. New insights in the immunologic basis of psoriasis. Seminars in Cutaneous Medicine and Surgery. 2010;**29**(1):3-9

[28] Chen Z, O'Shea JJ. Th17 cells: A new fate for differentiating helper T cells. Immunologic Research. 2008;**41**(2):87-102

[29] Fitzgerald O, Winchester R. Psoriatic arthritis: From pathogenesis to therapy. Arthritis Research & Therapy. 2009;**11**(1):214

[30] Mohan VK, Ganesan N, Gopalakrishnan R. Association of susceptible genetic markers and autoantibodies in rheumatoid arthritis. Journal of Genetics. 2014;**93**(2):597-605

[31] Rommel C, Camps M, Ji H. PI3K delta and PI3K gamma: Partners in crime in inflammation in rheumatoid arthritis and beyond? Nature Reviews. Immunology. 2007;7(3):191-201

[32] Castelino M, Barton A. Genetic susceptibility factors for psoriatic

arthritis. Current Opinion in Rheumatology. 2010;**22**(2):152-156

[33] O'Rielly DD, Rahman P. Genetics of psoriatic arthritis. Best Practice & Research. Clinical Rheumatology. 2014;**28**(5):673-685

[34] Yamamoto T. Psoriatic arthritis: From a dermatological perspective. European Journal of Dermatology. 2011;**21**(5):2011

[35] van Kuijk AW, Reinders-Blankert P, Smeets TJ, Dijkmans BA, Tak PP. Detailed analysis of the cell infiltrate and the expression of mediators of synovial inflammation and joint destruction in the synovium of patients with psoriatic arthritis: Implications for treatment. Annals of the Rheumatic Diseases 2006; 65 (12): 1551-1557

[36] Sabat R, Philipp S, Höflich C, Kreutzer S, Wallace E, Asadullah K, et al. Immunopathogenesis of psoriasis. Experimental Dermatology. 2007;**16**(10):779-798

[37] Belasco J, Louie JS, Gulati N, Wei N, Nograles K, Fuentes-Duculan J, et al. Comparative genomic profiling of synovium versus skin lesions in psoriatic arthritis. Arthritis & Rhematology. 2015;**67**(4):934-944

[38] Fitzgerald O, Haroon M, Giles JT, Winchester R. Concepts of pathogenesis in psoriatic arthritis: Genotype determines clinical phenotype. Arthritis Research & Therapy. 2015;**17**(1):115

[39] Firestein GS, Budd RC, Gabriel SE, et al. Kelley and Firestein's Textbook of Rheumatology. 10th ed. Vol. 2(10). Philadelphia, PA: Elsevier; 2017

[40] Janssen KMJ, de Smit MJ, Brouwer E, et al. Rheumatoid arthritis-associated autoantibodies in non-rheumatoid arthritis patients with mucosal inflammation: A case–control study. Arthritis Research & Therapy. 2015;**17**(1):174

[41] Coates LC, Helliwell PS. Psoriatic arthritis: State of the art review. Clinical Medicine. 2017;**17**(1):65-70

[42] Aletaha D, Neogi T, Silman AJ, et al. Rheumatoid arthritis classification criteria: An American College of Rheumatology/European league against rheumatism collaborative initiative. Arthritis and Rheumatism. 2010;**62**(9):2569-2581

[43] Scher JU, Ubeda C, Artacho A, et al. Decreased bacterial diversity characterizes the altered gut microbiota in patients with psoriatic arthritis, resembling dysbiosis in inflammatory bowel disease. Arthritis & Rhematology. 2015;**67**(1):128-139

[44] Helliwell PS, Hetthen J, Sokoll K, et al. Joint symmetry in early and late rheumatoid and psoriatic arthritis: Comparison with a mathematical model. Arthritis & Rheumatism. 2000;**42**(4):865-871

[45] Joaquim AF, Appenzeller S. Cervical spine involvement in rheumatoid arthritis—A systematic review. Autoimmunity Reviews. 2014;**13**:1195-1202

[46] Schett G, Lories RJ, D'Agostino M-A, et al. Enthesitis: From pathophysiology to treatment. Nature Reviews Rheumatology. 2017;**13**(12):731-741

[47] Krüger K, Burmester GR, Wassenberg S, et al. THU0141 A non-interventional clinical study evaluating the use of golimumab in patients with rheumatoid arthritis (RA), psoriatic arthritis (PSA), and ankylosing spondylitis (AS) in a real-life setting in Germany. Annals of the Rheumatic Diseases. 2016;**75**(2):1763

[48] Van der Horst-Bruinsma IE, Lems WF, Dijkmans BA. A systematic comparison of rheumatoid arthritis and ankylosing spondylitis. Clinical and Experimental Rheumatology. 2009;**27**(4):43-49

[49] Zlatanović G, Veselinović D, Cekić S, et al. Ocular manifestation of rheumatoid arthritis-different forms and frequency. Bosnian Journal of Basic Medical Sciences. 2010;**10**(4):323-327

[50] Shin D, Kim HJ, Kim DS, et al. Clinical features of psoriatic arthritis in Korean patients with psoriasis: A cross-sectional observational study of 196 patients with psoriasis using psoriatic arthritis screening questionnaires. Rheumatology International. 2016;**36**:207-212

[51] Wilson FC, Icen M, Crowson CS, et al. Incidence and clinical predictors of psoriatic arthritis in patients with psoriasis: A population-based study. Arthritis & Rheumatism. 2009;**61**(2):233-239

[52] Nishimura K, Sugiyama D, Kogata Y, Tsuji G, Nakazawa T, Kawano S, et al. Meta-analysis: Diagnostic accuracy of anti-cyclic citrullinated peptide antibody and rheumatoid factor for rheumatoid arthritis. Annals of Internal Medicine. 2007;**146**(11):797-808

[53] Eriksson C, Engstrand S, Sundqvist K-G, Rantapää-Dahlqvist S. Autoantibody formation in patients with rheumatoid arthritis treated with anti-TNFa. Annals of the Rheumatic Diseases. 2005;**64**(3):403-407

[54] Villani AP, Rouzaud M, Sevrain M, Barnetche T, Paul C, Richard MA, et al. Prevalence of undiagnosed psoriatic arthritis among psoriasis patients: Systematic review and meta-analysis. Journal of the American Academy of Dermatology. 2015;**73**(3):242-248

[55] Tucker LJ, Coates LC, Helliwell PS. Assessing disease activity in psoriatic arthritis: A literature review. Rheumatology and Therapy. 2019;**6**(1):23-32

[56] Armstrong EJ, Harskamp CT, Armstrong AW. Psoriasis and major adverse cardiovascular events: A systematic review and meta-analysis of observational studies. Journal of the American Heart Association. 2013;**2**(2):e000062

[57] Solomon DH, Goodson NJ, Katz JN, Weinblatt ME, Avorn J, Setoguchi S, et al. Patterns of cardiovascular risk in rheumatoid arthritis. Annals of the Rheumatic Diseases. 2006;**65**(12):1608-1612

[58] Lindhardsen J, Ahlehoff O, Gislason GH, Madsen OR, Olesen JB, Svendsen JH, et al. Risk of atrial fibrillation and stroke in rheumatoid arthritis: Danish nationwide cohort study. British Medical Journal. 2012;**344**:e1257

[59] Maradit-Kremers H, Nicola PJ, Crowson CS, Ballman KV, Gabriel SE. Cardiovascular death in rheumatoid arthritis: A population-based study. Arthritis and Rheumatism. 2005;**52**(3):722-732

[60] Gladman DD, Ang M, Su L, Tom BD, Schentag CT, Farewell VT. Cardiovascular morbidity in psoriatic arthritis. Annals of the Rheumatic Diseases. 2009;**68**(7):1131-1135

[61] Mellemkjaer L, Linet MS, Gridley G, Frisch M, Moller H, Olsen JH. Rheumatoid arthritis and cancer risk. European Journal of Cancer. 1996;**32**(10):1753-1757

[62] Chen YJ, Wu CY, Chen TJ, Shen JL, Chu SY, Wang CB, et al. The risk of cancer in patients with psoriasis: A population-based cohort study in Taiwan. Journal of the American Academy of Dermatology. 2011;**65**(1):84-91

[63] Marcil I, Stern RS. Squamous-cell cancer of the skin in patients given PUVA and ciclosporin: Nested cohort crossover study. Lancet. 2001;**358**(9287):1042-1045

[64] Rohekar S, Tom BD, Hassa A, Schentag CT, Farewell VT, Gladman DD. Prevalence of malignancy in psoriatic arthritis. Arthritis and Rheumatism. 2008;**58**(1):82-87

[65] Wong K, Gladman DD, Husted J, Long JA, Farewell VT. Mortality studies in psoriatic arthritis: Results from a single outpatient clinic. I. Causes and risk of death. Arthritis and Rheumatism. 1997;**40**(10):1868-1872

[66] Angulo P. Nonalcoholic fatty liver disease. The New England Journal of Medicine. 2002;**346**(16):1221-1231

[67] Ruderman EM, Crawford JM, Maier A, Liu JJ, Gravallese EM, Weinblatt ME. Histologic liver abnormalities in an autopsy series of patients with rheumatoid arthritis. British Journal of Rheumatology. 1997;**36**(2):210-213

[68] Miele L, Vallone S, Cefalo C, La Torre G, Di Stasi C, Vecchio FM, et al. Prevalence, characteristics and severity of non-alcoholic fatty liver disease in patients with chronic plaque psoriasis. Journal of Hepatology. 2009;**51**(4):778-786

[69] Nash P, Clegg DO. Psoriatic arthritis therapy: NSAIDs and traditional DMARDs. Annals of the Rheumatic Diseases. 2005;**64**(2):74-77

[70] Sarzi-Puttini P, Santandrea S, Boccassini L, Panni B, Caruso I. The role of NSAIDs in psoriatic arthritis: Evidence from a controlled study with nimesulide. Clinical and Experimental Rheumatology. 2001;**19**(1 Suppl. 22): 17-20

[71] Nas K, Karkucak M, Durmus B, et al. Comorbidities in patients with psoriatic arthritis: A comparison with rheumatoid arthritis and psoriasis. International Journal of Rheumatic Diseases. 2015;**18**(8):873-879

[72] Cañete JD, Pablos JL, Sanmartí R, et al. Antiangiogenic effects of anti-tumor necrosis factor α therapy with infliximab in psoriatic arthritis. Arthritis and Rheumatism. 2004;**50**(5):1636-1641

[73] Ortega C, Fernández-A S, Carrillo JM, et al. IL-17-producing CD8+ T lymphocytes from psoriasis skin plaques are cytotoxic. Effector cells that secrete Th17-related cytokines. Journal of Leukocyte Biology. 2009;**86**(2):435-443

[74] Mease PJ, van der Heijde D, Ritchlin CT, et al. Ixekizumab, an interleukin-17A specific monoclonal antibody, for the treatment of biologic-naive patients with active psoriatic arthritis: Results from the 24-week randomised, double-blind, placebo-controlled and active (adalimumab)-controlled period of the phase III trial SPIRIT-P1. Annals of the Rheumatic Diseases. 2017;**76**(1):79-87

[75] Stritesky GL, Yeh N, Kaplan MH. IL-23 promotes maintenance but not commitment to the Th17 lineage. Journal of Immunology. 2008;**181**(9):5948-5955

[76] Kavanaugh A, Puig L, Gottlieb AB, et al. Maintenance of clinical efficacy and radiographic benefit through two years of ustekinumab therapy in patients with

active psoriatic arthritis: Results from a randomized, placebo-controlled phase III trial. Arthritis Care and Research. 2015;**67**(12):1739-1749

[77] Deodhar A, Gottlieb A, Boehncke WH, et al. Efficacy and safety results of guselkumab, an anti-il23 monoclonal antibody, in patients with active psoriatic arthritis over 24 weeks: A phase 2a, randomized, double-blind, placebo-controlled study [abstract]. Annals of the Rheumatic Diseases. 2017;**76**(2):142-143

[78] Mease PJ, Kellner H, Morita A. Efficacy and safety results from a phase 2 trial of risankizumab, a selective IL-23p19 inhibitor, in patients with active psoriatic arthritis [abstract]. Arthritis and Rheumatism. 2017;**69**(10): Abstract 2L

[79] Rooney M, Symons JA, Duff GW. Interleukin 1 beta in synovial fluid is related to local disease activity in rheumatoid arthritis. Rheumatology International. 1990;**10**(5):217-219

[80] Taylor W, Gladman D, Helliwell P, et al. Classification criteria for psoriatic arthritis: Development of new criteria from a large international study. Arthritis & Rheumatism. 2006;**54**(8):2665-2673

[81] Amina LE, Gamily MEI. Biological impact of curcumin on the healing of tempromandibular joint in experimentally induced arthritis. Journal of Oral and Maxillofacial Surgery, Medicine, and Pathology. 2021;**33**:260-266

[82] Skyvalidas DN, Mavropoulos A, Tsiogkas S, Dardiotis E, Liaskos C, Mamuris Z, et al. Curcumin mediates attenuation of pro-inflammatory interferon γ and interleukin 17 cytokine responses in psoriatic disease, strengthening its role as a dietary immunosuppressant. Nutrition Research. 2020;**75**:95-108

[83] Martin BR. Treatment of psoriatic arthritis with acupuncture, turmeric (Curcuma longa), sarsaparilla (Smilax officinalis) and vitamin D: A case report. Journal of Chiropractic Medicine Martin. 2020;**19**(3):194-200

[84] Manca ML, Lattuada D, Valentia D, Marelli O, Corradini C, Fernàndez-Busquets X, et al. Potential therapeutic effect of curcumin loaded hyalurosomes against inflammatory and oxidative processes involved in the pathogenesis of rheumatoid arthritis: The use of fibroblast-like synovial cells cultured in synovial fluid. European Journal of Pharmaceutics and Biopharmaceutics. 2019;**136**:84-92

[85] Wang Q, Ye C, Sun S, Li R, Shi X, Wang S, et al. Curcumin attenuates collagen-induced rat arthritis via anti-inflammatory and apoptotic effects. International Immunopharmacology. 2019;**72**:292-300

[86] Dewangan AK, Perumal Y, Pavurala N, Chopra K, Mazumder S. Preparation, characterization and anti-inflammatory effects of curcumin loaded carboxymethyl cellulose acetate butyrate nanoparticles on adjuvant induced arthritis in rats. Journal of Drug Delivery Science and Technology. 2017;**41**:269-279. DOI: 10.1016/j.jddst.2017.07.022

[87] Jeengar MK, Shrivastava S, Chandra Mouli Veeravalli S, VGM N, Sistla R. Amelioration of FCA induced arthritis on topical application of curcumin in combination with emu oil. Nutrition. 2016;**9**:955-964. DOI: 10.1016/j.nut.2016.02.009